W9-AYW-012

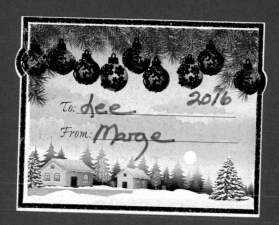

To: Lee   2016
From: Marge

Favorite Brand Name™
Gluten-Free

Publications International, Ltd.

Copyright © 2015 Publications International, Ltd.
All rights reserved. This publication may not be reproduced or quoted in whole or in part by any means whatsoever without written permission from:

Louis Weber, CEO
Publications International, Ltd.
7373 North Cicero Avenue
Lincolnwood, IL 60712

Permission is never granted for commercial purposes.

Favorite Brand Name is a trademark of Publications International, Ltd.

Recipe development on pages 218, 222, 224, 270 and 274 by Ellen Allard.
Recipe development on page 6 by Bev Bennett.
Recipe development on pages 148 and 158 by Marilyn Pocius.

Photography on pages 7, 149, 159, 219, 223, 225, 248, 253, 271, 275 and 279 by PIL Photo Studio, Chicago.
Photographer: Annemarie Zelasko
Photographer's Assistant: Tony Favarula
Food Stylists: Kathy Aragaki, Carol Smoler
Assistant Food Stylists: Sara Cruz, Lissa Levy

Pictured on the front cover *(left to right):* Tomato Zucchini Focaccia *(page 252),* Bean Ragoût with Cilantro-Cornmeal Dumplings *(page 12)* and Strawberry Shortcake *(page 154).*
Pictured on the back cover *(left to right):* Neptune's Spaghetti Squash *(page 36),* Flourless Peanut Butter Cookies *(page 166)* and Turkey and Winter Squash Tacos *(page 50).*

Contributing Writer: Marilyn Pocius

Photography on pages 104 and 105 by iStockphoto.

ISBN: 978-1-4508-9943-7

Library of Congress Control Number: 2011937417

Manufactured in China.

8 7 6 5 4 3 2 1

Microwave Cooking: Microwave ovens vary in wattage. Use the cooking times as guidelines and check for doneness before adding more time.

Note: This publication is only intended to provide general information. The information is specifically not intended to be a substitute for medical diagnosis or treatment by your physician or other health care professional. You should always consult your own physician or other health care professionals about any medical questions, diagnosis, or treatment. (Products vary among manufacturers. Please check labels carefully to confirm that the products you use are free of gluten.) **Not all recipes in this book are appropriate for all people with celiac disease, gluten intolerance, food allergies or sensitivities.**

The information obtained by you from this book should not be relied upon for any personal, nutritional, or medical decision. You should consult an appropriate professional for specific advice tailored to your specific situation. PIL makes no representations or warranties, express or implied, with respect to your use of this information.

In no event shall PIL, its affiliates or advertisers be liable for any direct, indirect, punitive, incidental, special, or consequential damages, or any damages whatsoever including, without limitation, damages for personal injury, death, damage to property, or loss of profits, arising out of or in any way connected with the use of any of the above-referenced information or otherwise arising out of the use of this book.

Publications International, Ltd.

Main Dishes
Contents

How to Eat Gluten-Free and Love it

What Is Gluten Anyway?

Gluten is a protein that is found in wheat, rye and barley. There are many reasons people avoid gluten. Celiac disease is the most serious. There are others who have a sensitivity to gluten and just feel better when they avoid it. Some people are allergic to wheat itself. You know which category you belong in if you're reading this book!

No More Bread? No Pasta?

At first, going gluten-free may sound awfully limiting. Fortunately, there are many more delicious foods on the gluten-free list than the forbidden list. There are also more and more products, from cereals to baking mixes to pastas, which are now being formulated in gluten-free versions. These days you'll find them not just in health food stores and online, but also on the shelves of most major supermarkets.

Some Good News

Spotting hidden gluten in processed foods is a lot easier now thanks to the FDA's Food Allergy Labeling Law that went into effect in 2004. Since wheat is a common allergen, any product that contains wheat or is derived from it must say so on the label. That means formerly questionable ingredients, such as modified food starch or maltodextrin, must now show wheat as part of their name if they were made from it (for example, "wheat maltodextrin"). Be aware that this ONLY applies to foods produced in the U.S. and Canada. Imports are a different matter.

More Good News

Look at your dietary restrictions as an opportunity to try new foods. Add quinoa and chickpea flour to your cupboard. Use corn tortillas to make sandwiches or lasagna. You'll find easy recipes in this book that are so delicious you'll forget that they're gluten-free. Healthy eating may actually be easier without gluten, too. Adding more fresh produce to your meals, eating less processed food and avoiding refined flour are all steps to a better diet for anyone.

The Short List

Sensitivities differ from person to person and ingredients differ from brand to brand. Always check the label's fine print. This is an abbreviated list of some of the most commonly used items.

•Red Lights• (contain gluten)	•Yellow Lights• (check ingredients)	•Green Lights• (no gluten)
barley	baking powder	beans
beer	barbecue sauce	buckwheat
bran	emulsifiers	cellophane noodles (bean thread noodles)
brewer's yeast	flavorings	
bulgur	frozen vegetables with sauce	chickpea flour (garbanzo flour)
cereal	marinades	corn, cornmeal
commercial baked goods	mustard	dairy
couscous	nondairy creamer	eggs
durum	oats*	fruit
graham	pasta sauce	lentils
gravies and sauces	salad dressings	meat & poultry
imitation seafood	soy sauce**	millet
kamut	vegetable broth	nuts
malt, malt flavoring and malt vinegar	*Most oats are processed in facilities that also handle wheat products. Look for oats processed in a dedicated gluten-free facility.	potatoes
matzo		quinoa
orzo		rice, rice flour
pizza		rice noodles
pretzels		seafood
rye	**Most soy sauce is brewed from soybeans and wheat. Look for brands that skip the brewing process and use soy concentrate and caramel coloring instead.	soy, soy flour
seitan		tapioca
semolina		tofu
spelt		vegetables (fresh, canned or frozen without sauce)
wheat		

Hot & Hearty

Chili-Topped Potato Boats

1 tablespoon canola oil

1 small onion, chopped

1 small green bell pepper, chopped

1 clove garlic, minced

1 pound ground beef

1 can (about 15 ounces) pinto or kidney beans, rinsed and drained

1 cup crushed tomatoes

1 tablespoon tomato paste

1 teaspoon chili powder

¾ teaspoon salt

½ teaspoon ground cumin

¼ teaspoon chipotle chile powder

¼ teaspoon black pepper

3 large baking potatoes, baked, halved lengthwise and scooped out

1. Heat oil in large nonstick skillet over medium heat. Add onion, bell pepper and garlic; cook and stir 5 to 6 minutes or until onion is tender. Add beef; brown 6 to 8 minutes, stirring to break up meat. Drain fat.

2. Stir in beans, tomatoes, tomato paste, chili powder, salt, cumin, chipotle chile powder and black pepper. Simmer 10 to 15 minutes or until mixture is hot and thick and flavors are blended. Spoon about ⅔ cup mixture into each potato half.

Makes 6 servings

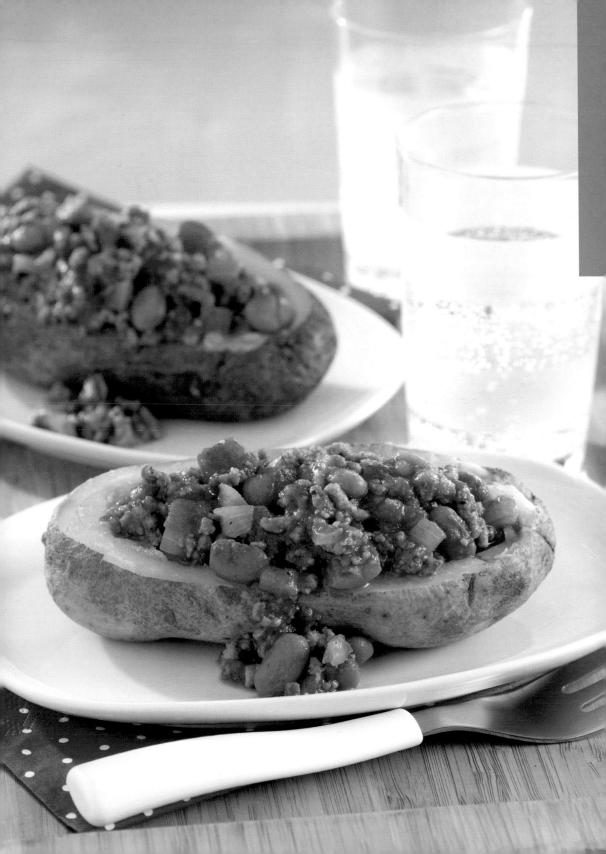

Bolognese-Style Pork Ragú
over Spaghetti Squash

1½ pounds ground pork
1 cup finely chopped celery
½ cup chopped onion
2 cloves garlic, minced
2 tablespoons tomato paste
1 teaspoon Italian seasoning
1 can (about 14 ounces) chicken broth
½ cup half-and-half
1 spaghetti squash (3 to 4 pounds)
½ cup grated Parmesan cheese (optional)

1. Brown pork in large saucepan over medium-high heat, stirring to break up meat. Add celery and onion; cook and stir over medium heat 5 minutes or until vegetables are tender. Add garlic; cook and stir 1 minute. Stir in tomato paste and Italian seasoning.

2. Stir in broth. Reduce heat. Simmer 10 to 15 minutes, stirring occasionally.

3. Add half-and-half; cook and stir until heated through. Skim off excess fat.

4. Meanwhile, pierce squash several times with knife. Microwave on HIGH 15 minutes or until squash is tender. Let cool slightly. Cut in half lengthwise; remove seeds. Separate strands with fork.

5. Serve meat sauce over squash. Sprinkle with cheese, if desired.

Makes 8 servings

Tip: Sauce can be cooked the day before and refrigerated so that chilled fat can be easily removed and discarded before reheating.

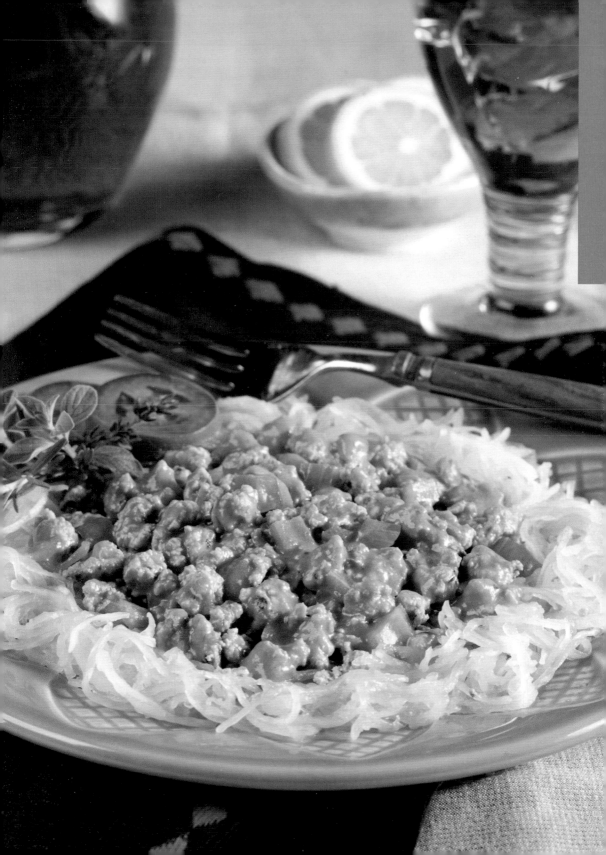

Roast Turkey Breast with Sausage and Apple Stuffing

....

8 ounces bulk pork sausage

1 medium apple, peeled and finely chopped

1 shallot or small onion, finely chopped

1 stalk celery, finely chopped

¼ cup chopped hazelnuts

½ teaspoon rubbed sage, divided

½ teaspoon salt, divided

½ teaspoon black pepper, divided

1 tablespoon butter, softened

1 whole boneless turkey breast (4½ to 5 pounds), thawed if frozen

4 to 6 fresh sage leaves (optional)

1 cup chicken broth

1. Preheat oven to 325°F. Crumble sausage into large skillet. Add apple, shallot and celery; cook and stir over medium-high heat until sausage is cooked through and apple and vegetables are tender. Drain fat. Stir in hazelnuts, ¼ teaspoon each sage, salt and pepper. Spoon stuffing into shallow roasting pan.

2. Combine butter and remaining ¼ teaspoon each sage, salt and pepper. Spread over turkey breast skin. (Arrange sage leaves under skin, if desired.) Place rack on top of stuffing. Place turkey, skin side down, on rack. Pour broth into pan.

3. Roast 45 minutes. Remove from oven; turn skin side up. Baste with broth; roast 1 hour or until meat thermometer registers 165°F. Remove from oven. Let turkey rest 10 minutes before carving.   *Makes 6 servings*

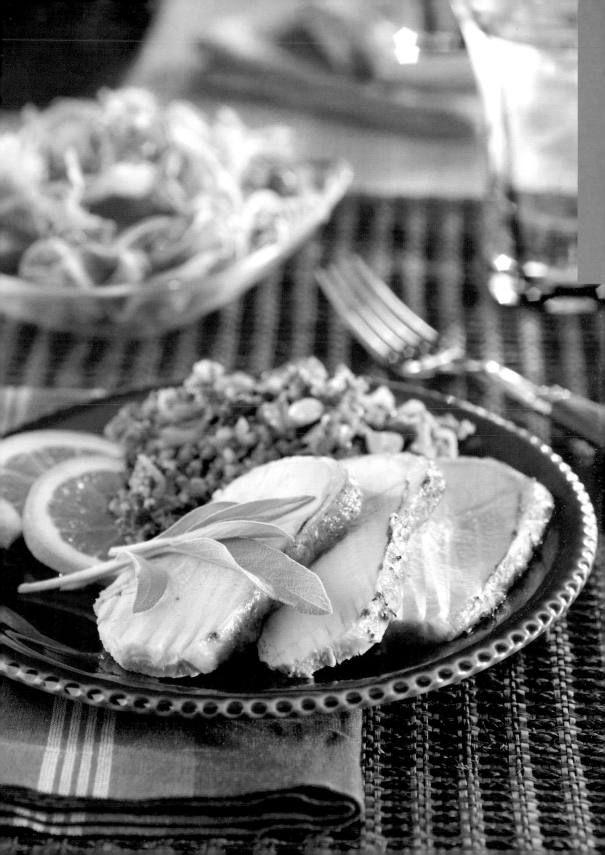

Bean Ragoût with Cilantro-Cornmeal Dumplings

· ·

1 tablespoon vegetable oil

2 large onions, chopped

1 poblano pepper, seeded and chopped

3 cloves garlic, minced

3 tablespoons chili powder

2 teaspoons ground cumin

1 teaspoon dried oregano

1 can (28 ounces) whole tomatoes, undrained, chopped

2 small zucchini, cut into ½-inch pieces

2 cups chopped red bell peppers

1 can (about 15 ounces) pinto beans, rinsed and drained

1 can (about 15 ounces) black beans, rinsed and drained

¾ teaspoon salt, divided

Black pepper

½ cup Gluten-Free All-Purpose Flour Blend (page 94)*

½ cup cornmeal

1 teaspoon baking powder

¼ teaspoon xanthan gum

2 tablespoons shortening

¼ cup (1 ounce) shredded Cheddar cheese

1 tablespoon minced fresh cilantro

½ cup milk

Or use any all-purpose gluten-free flour blend that does not contain xanthan gum.

1. Heat oil in Dutch oven over medium heat. Add onions; cook and stir 5 minutes or until tender. Add poblano pepper, garlic, chili powder, cumin and oregano; cook and stir 1 to 2 minutes.

2. Add tomatoes, zucchini, bell peppers, beans and ¼ teaspoon salt; bring to a boil. Reduce heat to medium-low. Simmer 5 to 10 minutes or until zucchini is tender. Season with black pepper.

continued on page 14

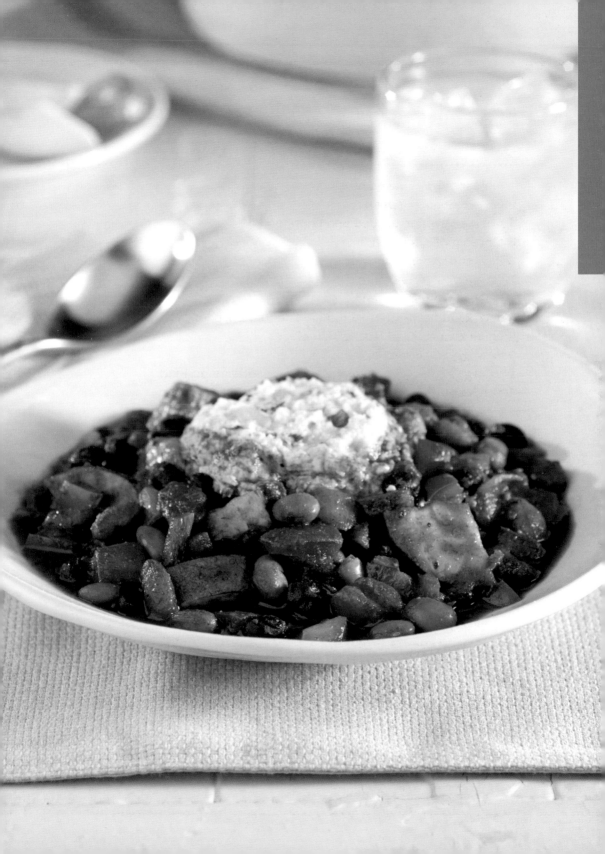

Bean Ragoût with Cilantro-Cornmeal Dumplings, continued

3. Meanwhile, prepare dumplings. Combine flour blend, cornmeal, baking powder, xanthan gum and remaining ½ teaspoon salt in medium bowl. Cut in shortening with pastry blender or two knives until mixture resembles coarse crumbs. Stir in cheese and cilantro. Add milk; stir just until dry ingredients are moistened.

4. Drop dumpling dough into 6 mounds on top of simmering ragoût. Cook, uncovered, 5 minutes. Cover; cook 5 to 10 minutes or until toothpick inserted into dumpling comes out clean. *Makes 6 servings*

Grilled Steak with Arugula & Gorgonzola Salad

4 boneless beef top loin (strip) steaks (¾ inch thick)
1 cup balsamic or red wine vinaigrette, divided
2 cups mixed salad greens
1½ cups baby arugula leaves
½ cup crumbled Gorgonzola* cheese

*Despite the fact that Gorgonzola (and other blue cheese) is sometimes made with a mold that can be derived from bread, recent studies have shown that it is safe. Even if the starter contains wheat, the gluten remaining in the finished product is practically undetectable.

1. Combine steaks and ½ cup vinaigrette in large resealable food storage bag. Seal bag; turn to coat. Marinate in refrigerator 20 to 30 minutes. Meanwhile, prepare grill for direct cooking.

2. Remove steaks from marinade; discard marinade. Place steaks on grid over medium-high heat. Grill, covered, 6 to 8 minutes for medium-rare (145°F) or until desired doneness, turning once.

3. Meanwhile, combine salad greens and arugula in medium bowl. Pour remaining ½ cup vinaigrette over greens; toss until well coated. Serve steaks with salad. Sprinkle with cheese. *Makes 4 servings*

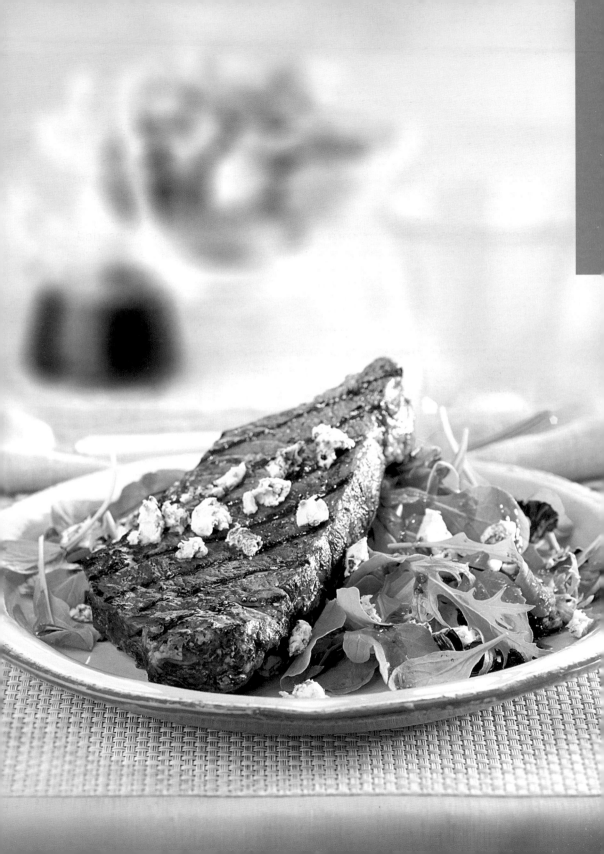

Baked Ham with Sweet and Spicy Glaze

1 (8-pound) bone-in smoked half ham
Sweet and Spicy Glaze (recipe follows)

1. Preheat oven to 325°F. Place ham, fat side up, on rack in roasting pan. Insert meat thermometer into thickest part of ham away from fat or bone. Roast about 3 hours.

2. Prepare Sweet and Spicy Glaze. Remove ham from oven. Generously brush half of glaze over ham; roast 30 minutes or until meat thermometer registers 160°F. Remove ham from oven; brush with remaining glaze. Let ham stand about 20 minutes before slicing.   *Makes 8 to 10 servings*

Sweet and Spicy Glaze

¾ **cup packed brown sugar**
⅓ **cup cider vinegar**
¼ **cup golden raisins**
1 **can (8¾ ounces) sliced peaches in heavy syrup, drained, chopped and syrup reserved**
1 **tablespoon cornstarch**
¼ **cup orange juice**
1 **can (8¾ ounces) crushed pineapple in syrup, undrained**
1 **tablespoon grated orange peel**
1 **clove garlic, minced**
½ **teaspoon red pepper flakes**
½ **teaspoon grated fresh ginger**

1. Combine brown sugar, vinegar, raisins and peach syrup in medium saucepan. Bring to a boil over high heat. Reduce heat to low; simmer 8 to 10 minutes.

2. Dissolve cornstarch in orange juice in small bowl; add to brown sugar mixture. Add remaining ingredients; mix well. Cook over medium heat, stirring constantly, until mixture boils and thickens.   *Makes about 2 cups*

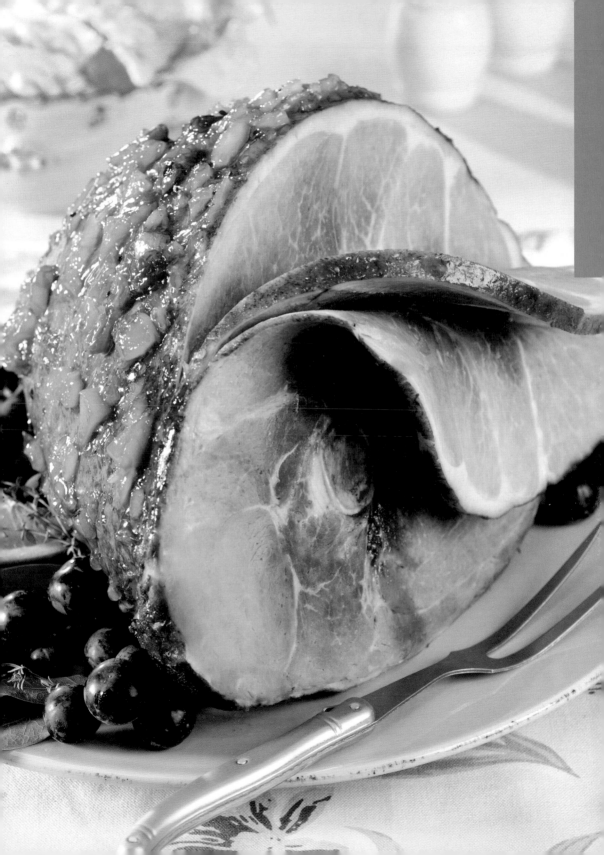

Family-Style Frankfurters with Rice and Red Beans

1 tablespoon vegetable oil

1 onion, chopped

½ green bell pepper, chopped

2 cloves garlic, minced

1 can (about 15 ounces) red kidney beans, rinsed and drained

1 can (about 15 ounces) Great Northern beans, rinsed and drained

½ pound gluten-free frankfurters, cut into ¼-inch-thick pieces

1 cup uncooked instant brown rice

1 cup chicken broth

¼ cup packed brown sugar

¼ cup ketchup

3 tablespoons dark molasses

1 tablespoon Dijon mustard

1. Preheat oven to 350°F. Lightly coat 13×9-inch baking dish with nonstick cooking spray.

2. Heat oil in Dutch oven over medium-high heat. Add onion, bell pepper and garlic; cook and stir 2 minutes or until tender.

3. Add beans, frankfurters, rice, broth, brown sugar, ketchup, molasses and mustard; stir to blend. Transfer to prepared baking dish.

4. Cover tightly with foil; bake 30 minutes or until rice is tender.

Makes 6 servings

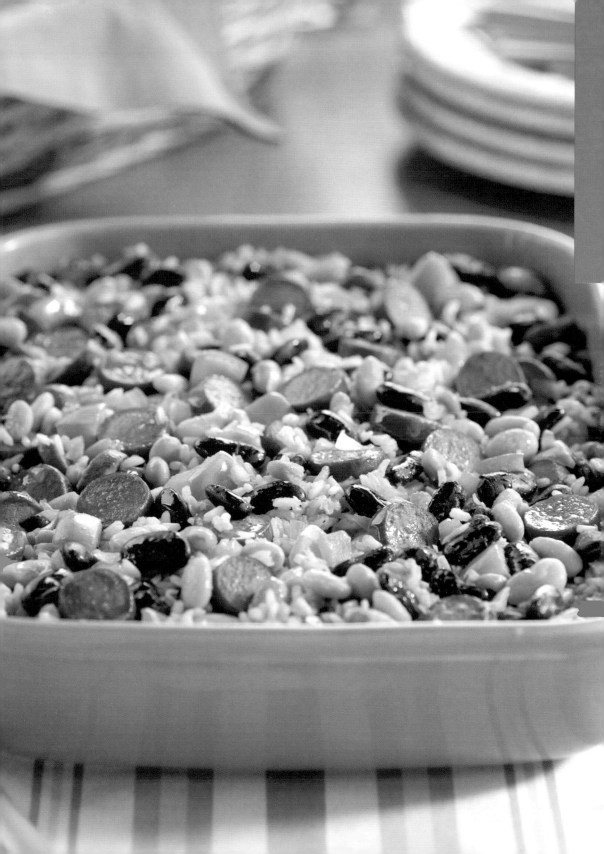

Summer Fiesta Casserole

2 pounds ground beef
1 medium onion, chopped
1 package (about 1 ounce) gluten-free taco seasoning
4 to 6 potatoes, cut into ½-inch cubes (about 4 cups)
1 to 2 tablespoons vegetable oil
4 cups sliced zucchini
1 can (about 14 ounces) diced tomatoes with onion and garlic
1½ cups (6 ounces) shredded Mexican cheese blend

1. Preheat oven to 350°F. Spray 4-quart casserole with nonstick cooking spray.

2. Cook beef and onion in large skillet over medium heat until meat is no longer pink, stirring to break up meat. Drain fat. Add taco seasoning and cook 5 minutes, stirring occasionally. Transfer to prepared casserole.

3. Add potatoes to same skillet; cook and stir over medium heat until potatoes are browned, adding oil as needed to prevent sticking. Add zucchini; cook and stir until beginning to soften. Transfer to casserole; top with tomatoes and cheese.

4. Bake 10 to 15 minutes or until cheese is melted and casserole is heated through. *Makes 4 to 6 servings*

Tip

Always check ingredient labels on spice mixes before using them. Most taco seasoning is free from gluten, but not all of it is. Check every time you purchase, even if you're buying the same brand, since formulations change frequently.

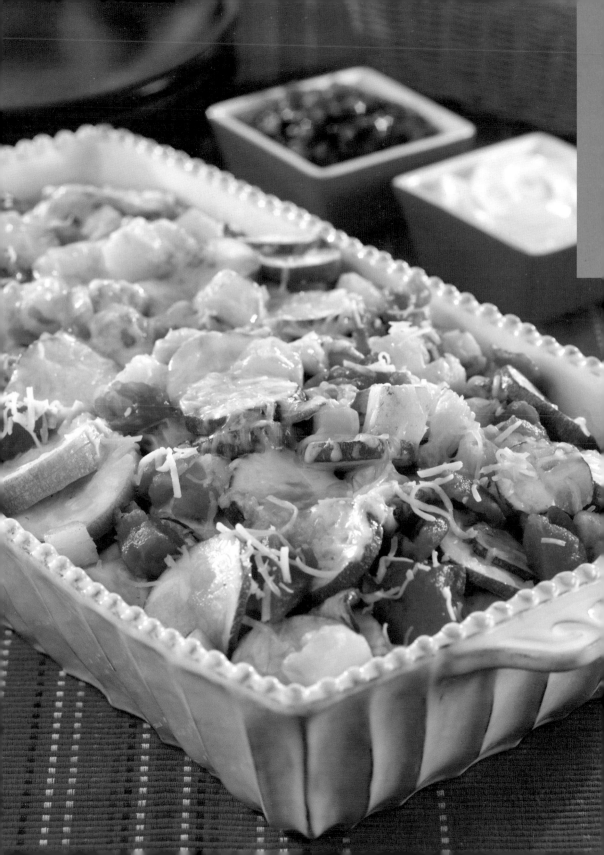

Bodacious Grilled Ribs

2 tablespoons paprika

2 teaspoons dried basil

½ teaspoon onion powder

¼ teaspoon garlic powder

¼ teaspoon ground red pepper

¼ teaspoon black pepper

4 pounds pork baby back ribs, cut into 4- to 6-rib pieces

8 ice cubes

1 cup gluten-free barbecue sauce

½ cup apricot fruit spread

1. Prepare grill for direct cooking. Spray two 24×18-inch sheets of heavy-duty foil with nonstick cooking spray.

2. Combine paprika, basil, onion powder, garlic powder, red pepper and black pepper in small bowl. Rub on both sides of ribs. Place 2 pounds of ribs in single layer in center of each foil sheet. Place 4 ice cubes on top of each.

3. Double-fold sides and ends of foil to seal packets, leaving head space for heat circulation.

4. Transfer packets to grid. Grill over medium heat, covered, 45 to 60 minutes or until tender. Carefully open one end of each packet to allow steam to escape.

5. Combine barbecue sauce and fruit spread in small bowl. Transfer ribs to grid. Brush with barbecue sauce mixture. Grill 5 to 10 minutes, brushing with sauce and turning often.

Makes 4 servings

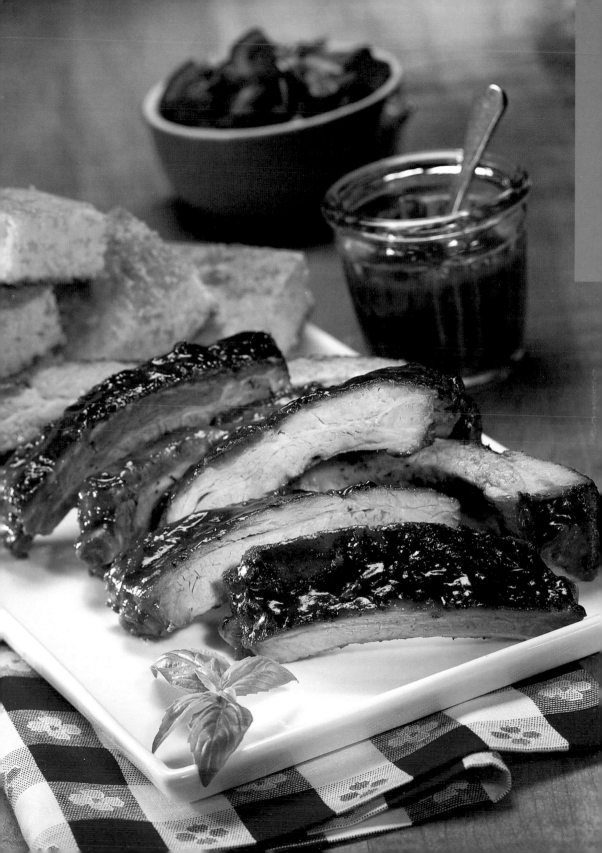

Mexican Lasagna

1 pound ground beef
1 package (about 1 ounce) gluten-free taco seasoning
1 can (about 14 ounces) Mexican-style diced tomatoes
1½ teaspoons chili powder
1 teaspoon ground cumin
½ teaspoon salt
½ teaspoon red pepper flakes
2 cups (16 ounces) sour cream
1 can (4 ounces) diced mild green chiles, drained
6 green onions, chopped
6 (6-inch) corn tortillas
1 can (15 ounces) corn, drained
2 cups (8 ounces) shredded Cheddar cheese

1. Preheat oven to 350°F. Grease 4-quart casserole.

2. Cook ground beef with taco seasoning in large skillet over medium heat until meat is no longer pink, stirring to break up meat. Drain fat.

3. Combine tomatoes, chili powder, cumin, salt and red pepper flakes in medium bowl.

4. Combine sour cream, chiles and green onions in small bowl.

5. Layer one third of tomato mixture, 2 tortillas, one third of sour cream mixture, one third of meat mixture, one third of corn and one third of cheese in prepared casserole. Repeat layers twice.

6. Bake 35 minutes or until bubbly. Let stand 15 minutes before serving.

Makes 4 servings

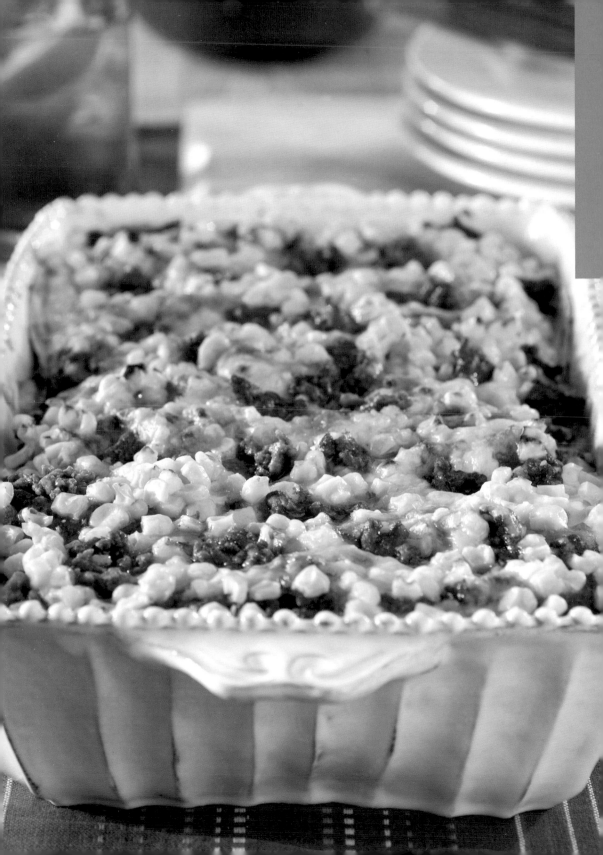

Pork Curry over Cauliflower Couscous

3 tablespoons olive oil, divided
2 tablespoons mild curry powder
2 teaspoons minced garlic
1½ pounds boneless pork, cubed
1 red or green bell pepper, diced
1 tablespoon cider vinegar
½ teaspoon salt
2 cups water
1 large head cauliflower

1. Heat 2 tablespoons oil in large saucepan over medium heat. Add curry powder and garlic; cook and stir 1 to 2 minutes or until garlic is golden.

2. Add pork; cook and stir 5 to 7 minutes or until pork cubes are barely pink in center. Add bell pepper and vinegar; cook and stir 3 minutes or until bell pepper is soft. Sprinkle with salt.

3. Add water; bring to a boil. Reduce heat and simmer 30 to 45 minutes or until liquid is reduced and pork is tender, stirring occasionally, adding additional water as needed.

4. Meanwhile, trim and core cauliflower; cut into equal pieces. Place in food processor. Process using on/off pulsing action until cauliflower is in small uniform pieces about the size of cooked couscous. *Do not purée.*

5. Heat remaining 1 tablespoon oil in large nonstick skillet over medium heat. Add cauliflower; cook and stir 5 minutes or until crisp-tender. *Do not overcook.* Serve pork curry over cauliflower. *Makes 6 servings*

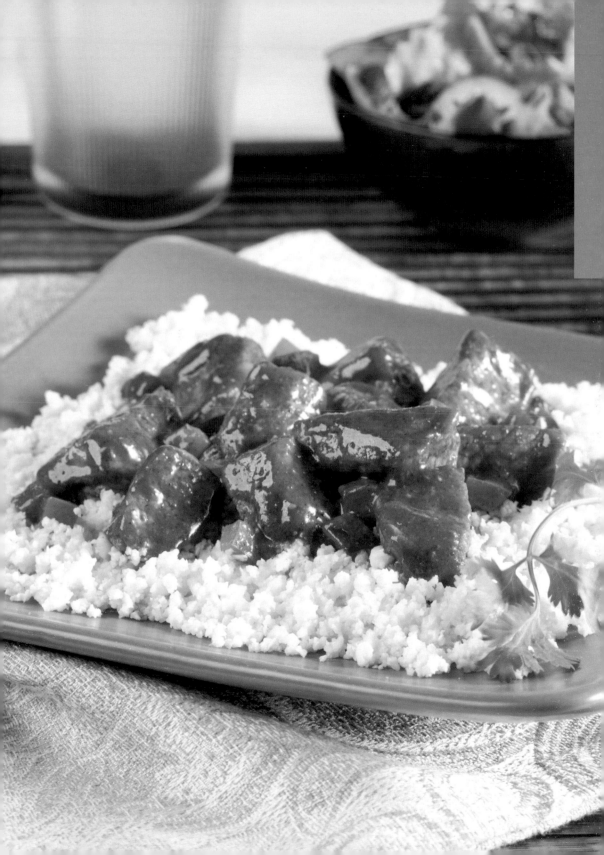

Savvy Seafood

Greek-Style Salmon

··

    2 teaspoons olive oil
1¾ cups diced tomatoes, drained
    6 pitted black olives, coarsely chopped
    4 pitted green olives, coarsely chopped
    3 tablespoons lemon juice
    2 tablespoons chopped fresh Italian parsley
    1 tablespoon capers, drained
    2 cloves garlic, thinly sliced
    ¼ teaspoon black pepper
    1 pound salmon fillets

1. Heat oil in large skillet over medium heat. Add tomatoes, olives, lemon juice, parsley, capers, garlic and pepper. Bring to a simmer, stirring frequently. Simmer 5 minutes or until reduced by about one third, stirring occasionally.

2. Rinse salmon and pat dry with paper towels. Push sauce to one side of skillet. Add salmon; spoon sauce over salmon. Cover and cook 10 to 15 minutes or until salmon begins to flake when tested with fork.

Makes 4 servings

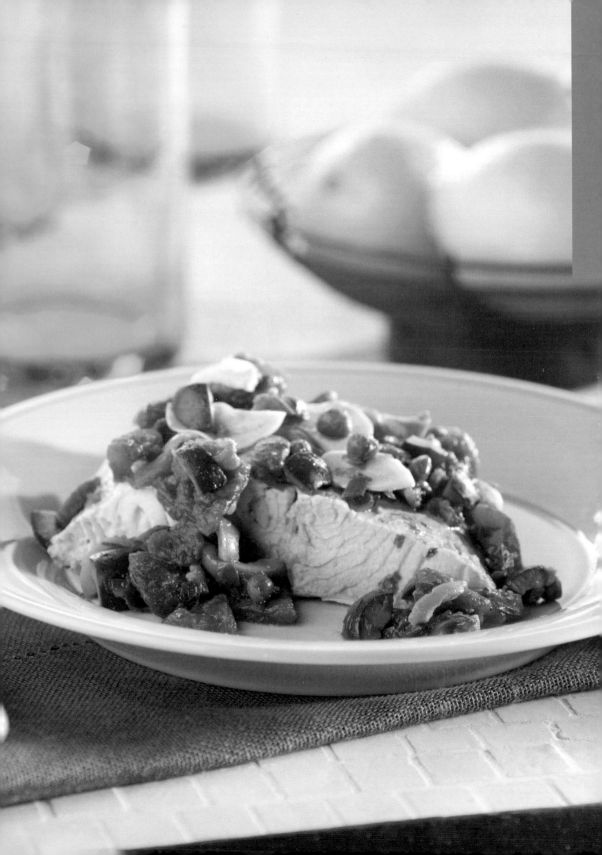

Cheesy Shrimp on Grits

1 cup finely chopped green bell pepper

1 cup finely chopped red bell pepper

¾ cup chopped green onions, divided

½ cup thinly sliced celery

¼ cup (½ stick) butter, cubed

1¼ teaspoons gluten-free seafood seasoning

2 bay leaves

¼ teaspoon ground red pepper

1 pound raw shrimp, peeled and deveined

1⅓ cups quick-cooking corn grits

2 cups (8 ounces) shredded sharp Cheddar cheese

¼ cup whipping cream or half-and-half

Slow Cooker Directions

1. Coat slow cooker with nonstick cooking spray. Add bell peppers, ¼ cup green onions, celery, butter, seafood seasoning, bay leaves and ground red pepper. Cover; cook on LOW 4 hours or on HIGH 2 hours.

2. *Turn slow cooker to HIGH.* Add shrimp. Cover; cook 15 minutes. Meanwhile, prepare grits according to package directions.

3. Remove and discard bay leaves from shrimp mixture. Stir in cheese, cream and remaining ½ cup green onions. Cook, uncovered, 5 minutes or until cheese melts. Serve over grits.   *Makes 6 servings*

Variation: This dish is also delicious served over polenta or quinoa.

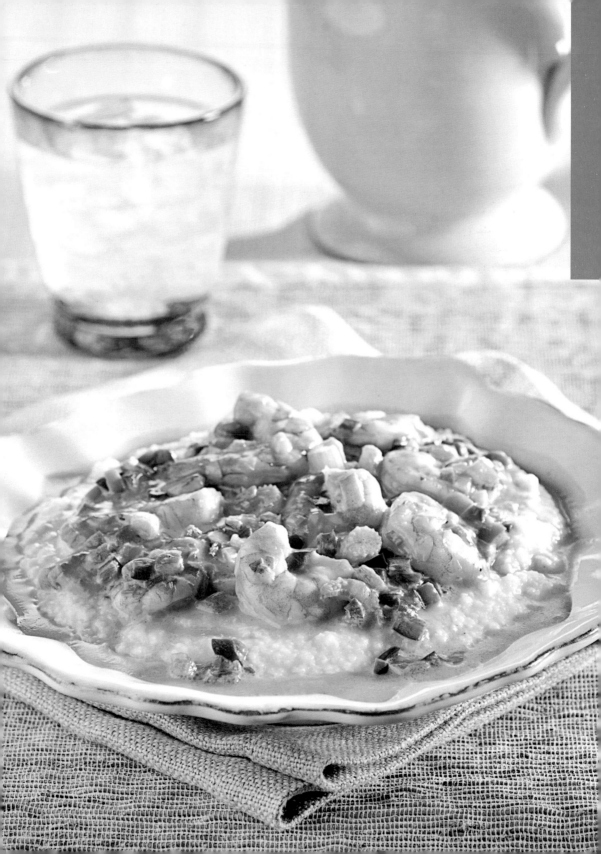

Pecan Catfish with Cranberry Compote

        Cranberry Compote (recipe follows)
1½ **cups pecans**
  2 **tablespoons rice flour**
  1 **egg**
  2 **tablespoons water**
     Salt and black pepper
  4 **catfish fillets (about 1¼ pounds)**
  2 **tablespoons butter, divided**

1. Prepare Cranberry Compote. Preheat oven to 425°F.

2. Place pecans and rice flour in food processor; process just until finely chopped. *Do not overprocess.* Place pecan mixture in shallow dish or plate. Whisk egg and water in another shallow dish. Sprinkle salt and pepper on both sides of each fillet; dip in egg mixture, then in pecan mixture, pressing to make coating stick.

3. Place 1 tablespoon butter in 13×9-inch baking pan. Melt butter on stovetop or in oven and tilt pan to distribute evenly. Place fillets in prepared pan in single layer. Dot with remaining 1 tablespoon butter.

4. Bake 15 to 20 minutes or until fish begins to flake when tested with fork. Serve with Cranberry Compote. *Makes 4 servings*

Cranberry Compote

  1 **package (12 ounces) cranberries**
¾ **cup water**
⅔ **cup sugar**
¼ **cup orange juice**
  2 **teaspoons grated fresh ginger**
¼ **teaspoon Chinese five-spice powder**
⅛ **teaspoon salt**
  1 **teaspoon butter**

continued on page 34

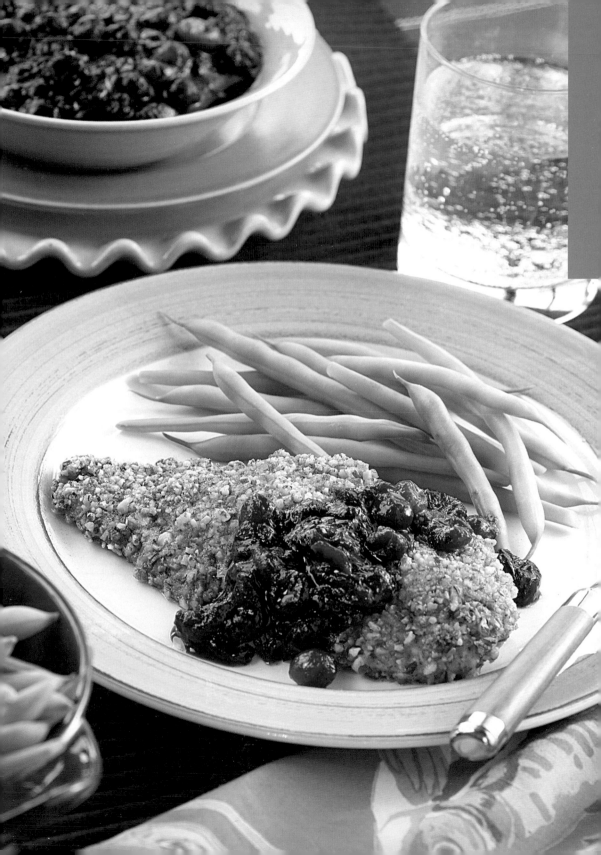

1. Combine cranberries, water, sugar, orange juice, ginger, five-spice powder and salt in large saucepan. Heat over medium-high heat 10 minutes or until berries begin to pop, stirring occasionally.

2. Cook and stir 5 minutes or until thickened. Remove from heat; stir in butter. Let stand 10 minutes; refrigerate until chilled. Compote can be made ahead and stored up to 1 week in refrigerator. *Makes about 3 cups*

Grilled Fish Tacos

  ¾ **teaspoon chili powder**
   1 **pound skinless mahi mahi, halibut or tilapia fillets**
  ½ **cup salsa, divided**
   2 **cups packaged coleslaw mix or shredded cabbage**
  ¼ **cup sour cream**
   4 **tablespoons chopped fresh cilantro, divided**
   8 **(6-inch) corn tortillas, warmed according to package directions**

1. Prepare grill for direct cooking. Sprinkle chili powder over fish. Spoon ¼ cup salsa over fish; let stand 10 minutes. Meanwhile, combine coleslaw mix, remaining ¼ cup salsa, sour cream and 2 tablespoons cilantro in large bowl; mix well.

2. Grill fish, salsa side up, over medium heat, covered, 8 to 10 minutes or until fish is opaque in center, without turning. Slice fish crosswise into thin strips or cut into chunks. Fill warm tortillas with fish and coleslaw mix. Garnish with remaining cilantro. *Makes 4 servings*

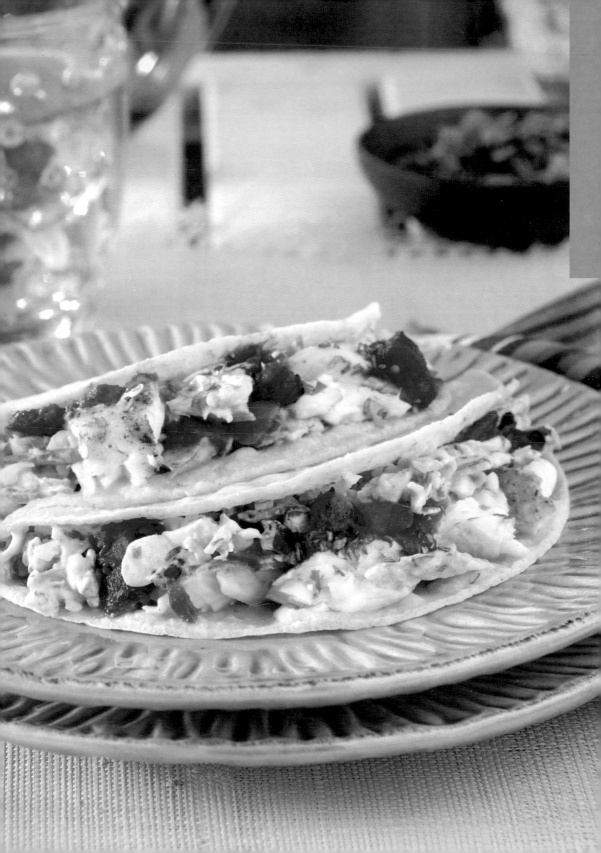

Neptune's Spaghetti Squash

1 **spaghetti squash (about 3 pounds)**
2 **tablespoons olive oil**
1 **clove garlic, minced**
½ **pound medium raw shrimp, peeled and deveined**
½ **pound bay scallops**
½ **cup fresh or frozen peas**
¼ **cup sun-dried tomatoes in oil, drained and chopped***
½ **teaspoon dried basil**
¼ **cup grated Parmesan cheese**

Or substitute 2 plum tomatoes, seeded and chopped, for sun-dried tomatoes.
(To seed tomatoes, cut in half. Remove seeds with spoon and discard.)

1. Preheat oven to 375°F. Line baking dish with foil.

2. Pierce squash in several places with knife. Place squash in prepared baking dish. Bake 20 minutes. Turn squash over; bake 25 minutes or until tender. Let cool slightly.

3. Meanwhile, heat oil in large skillet over medium-high heat. Cook and stir garlic 1 minute. Add shrimp, scallops, peas, tomatoes and basil; cook and stir 1 to 2 minutes or until shrimp turn pink and scallops are opaque. Keep warm.

4. Cut squash in half lengthwise; remove seeds. Separate strands with fork.

5. Top squash with seafood mixture; toss gently to coat. Sprinkle with cheese.

Makes 4 servings

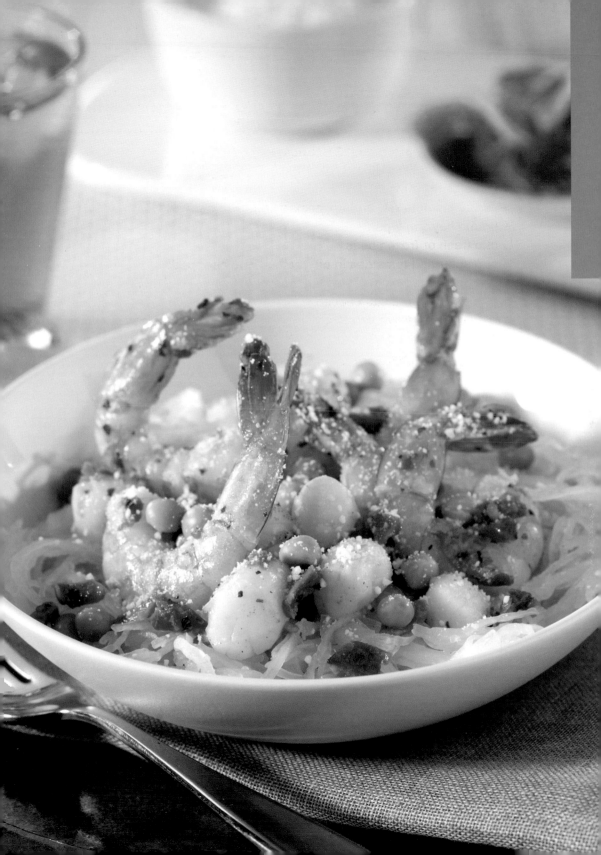

Crab and Corn Enchilada Casserole

Spicy Tomato Sauce (recipe follows), divided
10 to 12 ounces crabmeat, fresh, frozen or pasteurized
1 package (10 ounces) frozen corn, thawed and drained
1½ cups (6 ounces) shredded Monterey Jack cheese, divided
1 can (4 ounces) diced mild green chiles
12 (6-inch) corn tortillas
1 lime, cut into 6 wedges

1. Prepare Spicy Tomato Sauce. Preheat oven to 350°F. Pick out and discard any shell or cartilage from crabmeat.

2. Combine 2 cups Spicy Tomato Sauce, crabmeat, corn, 1 cup cheese and chiles in medium bowl. Cut each tortilla into 4 wedges. Place one third of tortilla wedges in shallow 3- to 4-quart casserole, overlapping to make solid layer. Spread half of crab mixture on top. Repeat with another layer of tortilla wedges, remaining crab mixture and remaining tortillas. Spread remaining 1 cup Spicy Tomato Sauce over top; cover.

3. Bake 30 to 40 minutes or until heated through. Sprinkle with remaining ½ cup cheese; bake, uncovered, 5 minutes or until cheese melts. Serve with lime wedges. *Makes 6 servings*

Spicy Tomato Sauce

2 cans (about 14 ounces each) stewed tomatoes, undrained
2 teaspoons olive oil
1 medium onion, chopped
1 tablespoon minced garlic
2 tablespoons chili powder
2 teaspoons ground cumin
2 teaspoons dried oregano
1 teaspoon ground cinnamon
¼ teaspoon *each* red pepper flakes and ground cloves

continued on page 40

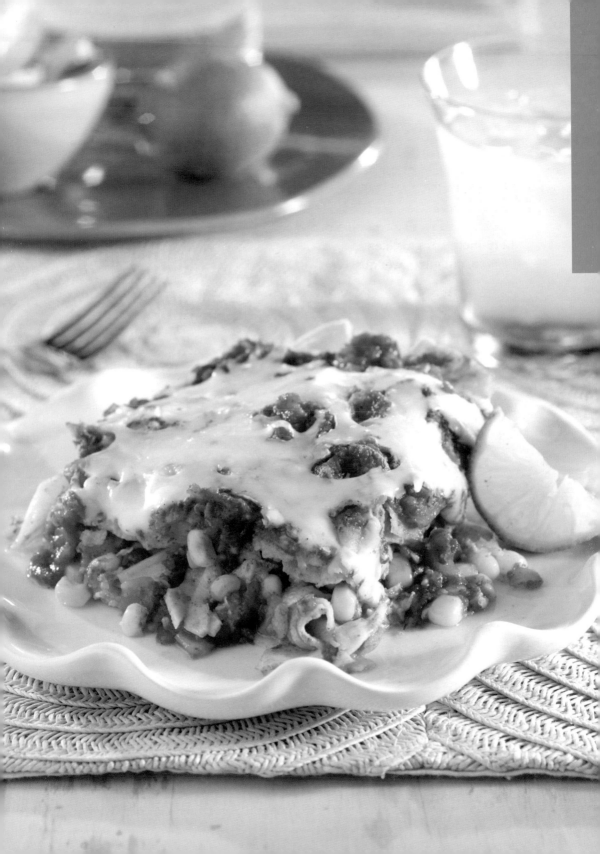

Spicy Tomato Sauce, continued

1. Place tomatoes in food processor or blender; process until finely chopped. Set aside.

2. Heat oil in large saucepan over medium-high heat. Add onion and garlic; cook and stir 5 minutes or until onion is tender. Add chili powder, cumin, oregano, cinnamon, red pepper flakes and cloves; cook and stir 1 minute. Add tomatoes; reduce heat to medium-low. Simmer, uncovered, 20 minutes or until sauce is reduced to about 3 cups. *Makes 3 cups*

Smoked Salmon Hash Browns

3 cups frozen hash brown potatoes, thawed
2 pouches (3 ounces each) smoked salmon*
½ cup chopped onion
½ cup chopped green bell pepper
¼ teaspoon black pepper
2 tablespoons vegetable oil

*Smoked salmon in foil pouches can be found in the canned fish section of the supermarket. Do not substitute lox or other fresh smoked salmon.

1. Combine potatoes, salmon, onion, bell pepper and black pepper in large bowl; mix well.

2. Heat oil in large skillet over medium-high heat. Add potato mixture; pat down evenly.

3. Cook 5 minutes or until bottom is crisp and brown. Turn over in large pieces. Cook 2 to 3 minutes or until both sides are browned.

Makes 4 servings

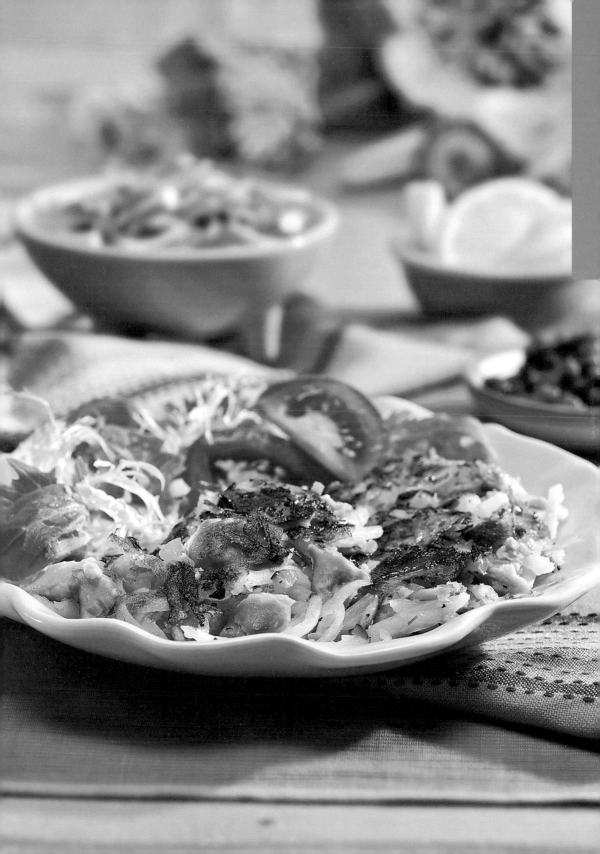

Grilled Tuna and Succotash Salad

⅔ **cup vegetable oil**

¼ **cup chopped fresh basil**

3 **tablespoons balsamic or red wine vinegar**

2 **tablespoons Dijon mustard**

2 **tablespoons lemon juice**

½ **teaspoon salt**

½ **teaspoon black pepper**

4 **tuna steaks (about 6 ounces each)**

2 **cups frozen baby lima beans, cooked according
      to package directions**

1 **cup frozen corn, thawed**

2 **large tomatoes, seeded and chopped**

   Arugula or spinach leaves

   Lemon slices and fresh dill sprigs (optional)

1. Whisk oil, basil, vinegar, mustard, lemon juice, salt and pepper in small bowl.

2. Rinse tuna and pat dry with paper towels. Place tuna in shallow glass dish. Pour ¾ cup oil mixture over tuna; turn to coat. Cover and refrigerate 30 minutes.

3. Prepare grill for direct cooking. Combine lima beans, corn and tomatoes in large bowl. Stir in remaining oil mixture. Cover and let stand at room temperature until ready to serve.

4. Drain tuna; discard marinade. Grill over medium-high heat 6 to 8 minutes or until desired doneness, turning halfway through grilling time.

5. Serve tuna on arugula. Spoon bean mixture over tuna. Garnish with lemon slices and dill.

Makes 4 servings

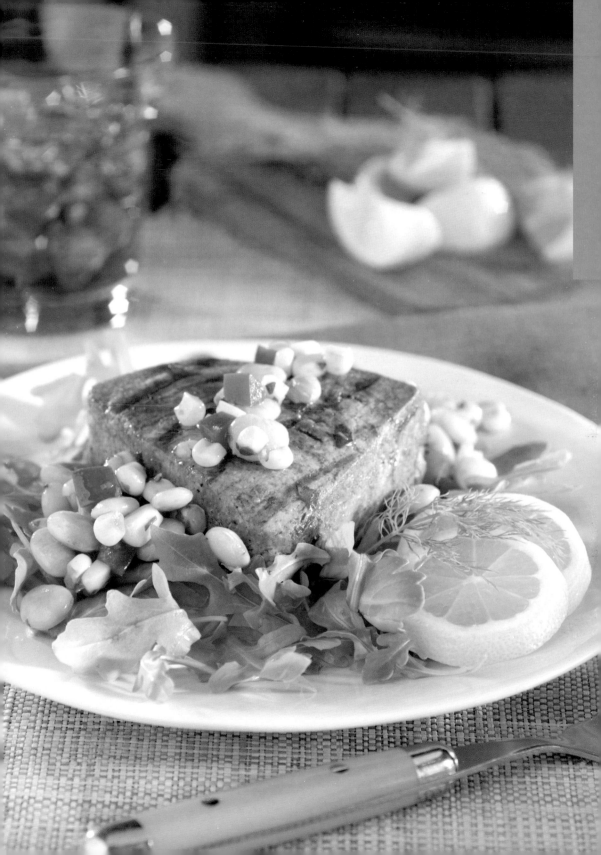

Asian Pesto Noodles

Spicy Asian Pesto (recipe follows), divided
1 pound large raw shrimp, peeled and deveined
12 ounces uncooked gluten-free noodles or spaghetti

1. Prepare Spicy Asian Pesto. Marinate shrimp in ¾ cup Pesto.

2. Cook noodles according to package directions; drain and set aside. Preheat broiler or grill.

3. Place marinated shrimp on metal skewers. (If using wooden skewers, soak in water for at least 30 minutes to prevent burning.) Place skewers under broiler or on grill; cook about 3 minutes per side or until shrimp are opaque.

4. To serve, toss noodles with remaining Pesto. Serve with shrimp.

Makes 4 servings

Spicy Asian Pesto

3 cups fresh basil leaves
3 cups fresh cilantro leaves
3 cups fresh mint leaves
¾ cup peanut oil
3 tablespoons sugar
2 to 3 tablespoons lime juice
5 cloves garlic, chopped
2 teaspoons fish sauce *or* 1 teaspoon salt
1 serrano pepper,* finely chopped

*Serrano peppers can sting and irritate the skin, so wear rubber gloves when handling peppers and do not touch your eyes.

Combine all ingredients in blender or food processor; blend until smooth.

Makes 2½ cups

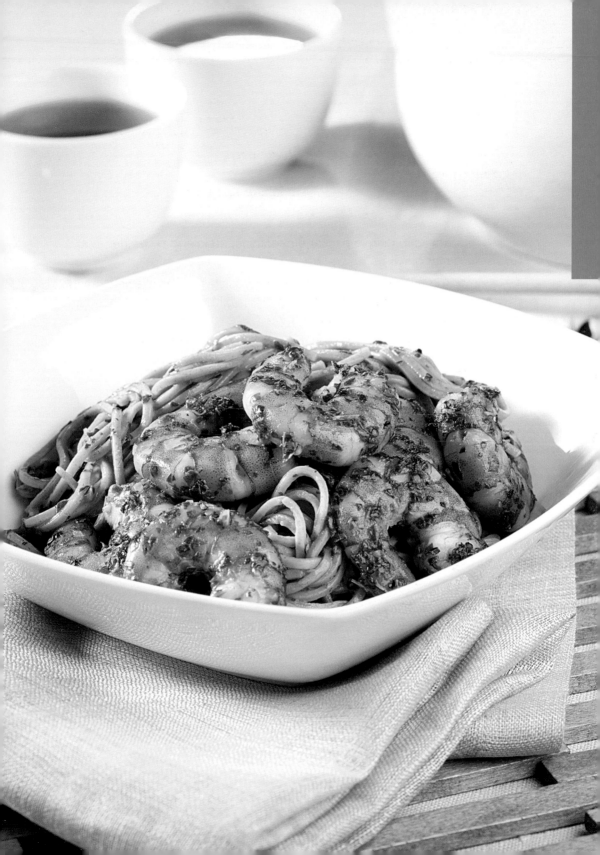

Better Birds

Honey-Roasted Chicken and Butternut Squash

1 pound fresh butternut squash chunks
Salt and black pepper
6 bone-in chicken thighs
1 tablespoon honey

1. Preheat oven to 375°F. Spray baking sheet and wire rack with nonstick cooking spray.

2. Spread squash on prepared baking sheet; season with salt and pepper.

3. Place wire rack over squash; place chicken on rack. Season with salt and pepper.

4. Roast 25 minutes. Carefully lift rack and stir squash; brush honey over chicken pieces. Roast 20 minutes or until chicken is cooked through (165°F).

Makes 4 to 6 servings

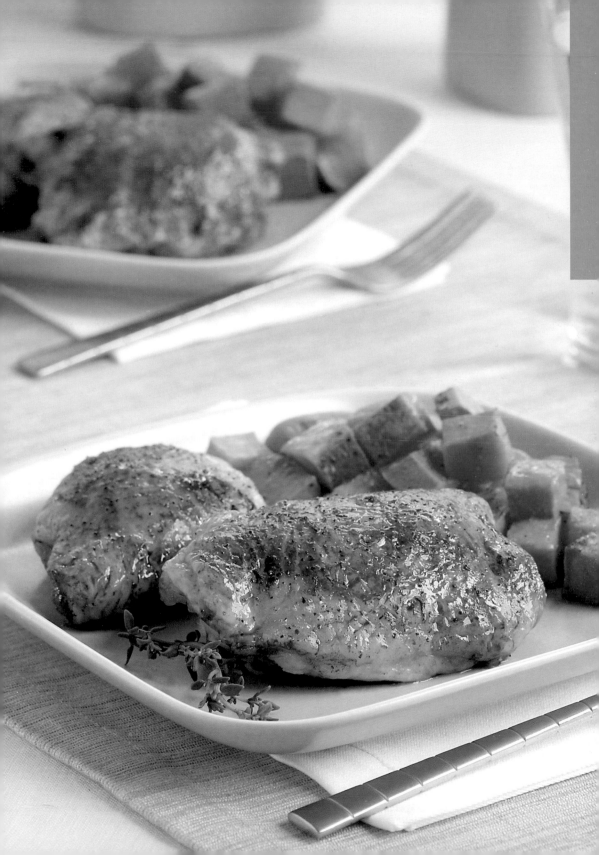

Greek Chicken Burgers with Cucumber Yogurt Sauce

1¼ cups Greek yogurt

1 medium cucumber, peeled, seeded and finely chopped

4 cloves garlic, minced, divided

1 tablespoon minced fresh mint

Juice of 1 lemon

¼ teaspoon salt

⅛ teaspoon white pepper

1 pound ground chicken

3 ounces crumbled feta cheese

4 large kalamata olives, minced

½ to 1 teaspoon dried oregano

¼ teaspoon black pepper

1 egg

1. Mix yogurt, cucumber, 3 minced garlic cloves, mint, lemon juice, salt and white pepper in medium bowl. Refrigerate until ready to serve.

2. Combine chicken, feta, olives, oregano, black pepper and remaining garlic in large bowl; blend well.

3. Beat egg in small bowl. Add to chicken mixture; blend thoroughly. Form into 4 patties.

4. Coat grill pan with nonstick cooking spray; heat over medium-high heat. Grill burgers 5 to 7 minutes per side or until cooked through (165°F).

5. Serve burgers with cucumber yogurt sauce. *Makes 4 servings*

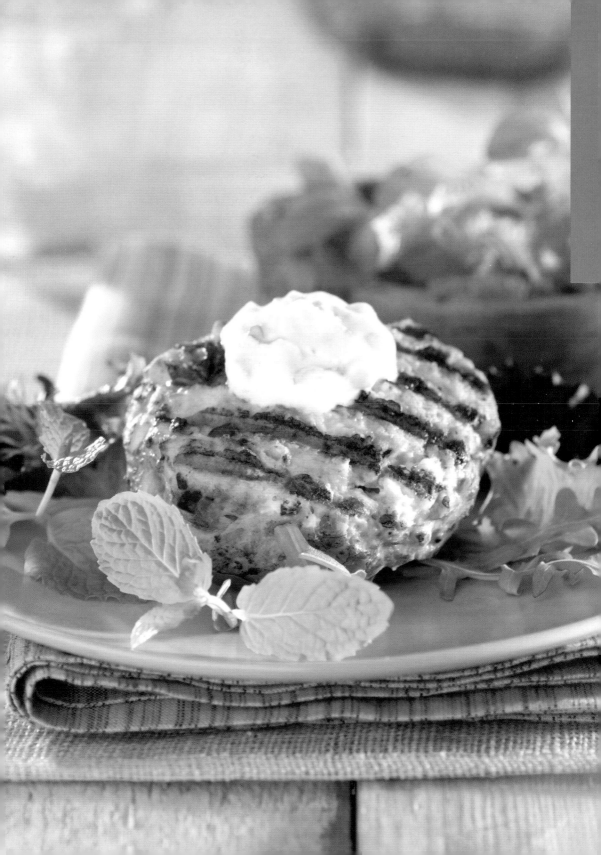

Turkey and Winter Squash Tacos

4 crisp corn taco shells
2 teaspoons vegetable oil
¼ cup finely chopped onion
1 cup diced cooked butternut or delicata squash (see Note)
1 teaspoon gluten-free taco seasoning
1 cup chopped cooked turkey, warmed
Salt and black pepper
¼ cup salsa
1 avocado, cut into 8 thin wedges

1. Preheat oven to 325°F. Place taco shells on baking sheet; heat according to package directions.

2. Meanwhile, heat oil in large skillet over medium-high heat. Add onion; cook and stir 3 minutes. Add squash and taco seasoning; cook and stir 2 to 3 minutes.

3. To assemble tacos, place ¼ cup turkey in each taco shell. Season with salt and pepper. Top with squash mixture, salsa and avocado.

Makes 2 servings

Note: Some supermarkets carry packaged diced squash; simply follow the cooking instructions on the package. To use whole squash, peel the squash, cut in half and remove the seeds. Cut the squash into ¾-inch-long strips, then cut crosswise into ¾-inch chunks. Measure 1 cup squash. Heat 1 tablespoon vegetable oil in a medium skillet over medium-low heat. Add the squash; cook and stir 10 to 15 minutes or until fork-tender.

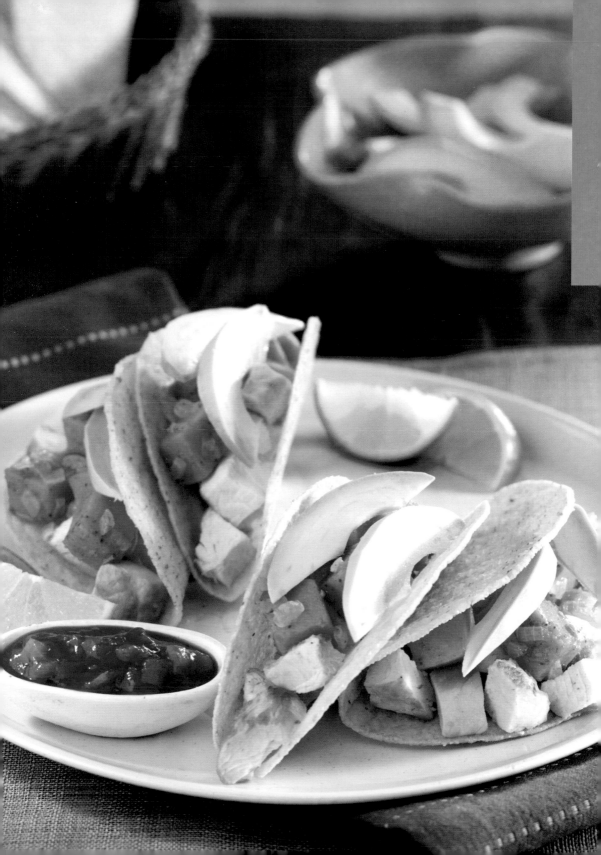

Flourless Fried Chicken Tenders

1½ cups chickpea flour*
1½ teaspoons Italian seasoning
1 teaspoon salt
½ teaspoon black pepper
⅛ teaspoon ground red pepper
¾ cup plus 2 to 4 tablespoons water
Oil for frying
1 pound chicken tenders, cut in half if large
Curry Mayo Dipping Sauce (recipe follows, optional)

*Chickpea flour is also called garbanzo flour. It is found in the specialty flour section of most supermarkets.

1. Sift chickpea flour into medium bowl. Stir in Italian seasoning, salt, black pepper and red pepper. Gradually whisk in ¾ cup water to make smooth batter. Whisk in additional water by tablespoons if needed until batter is consistency of heavy cream.

2. Meanwhile, add oil to large heavy skillet or Dutch oven to ¾-inch depth. Heat over medium-high heat until drop of batter placed in oil sizzles (350°F).

3. Pat chicken pieces dry. Dip pieces into batter with tongs; let excess fall back into bowl. Ease chicken gently into oil; fry 2 to 3 minutes per side or until slightly browned and chicken is cooked through. Fry in batches and do not crowd pan.

4. Drain chicken on paper towels. Serve warm with Curry Mayo Dipping Sauce, if desired.   *Makes 4 servings*

Curry Mayo Dipping Sauce: Combine ½ cup mayonnaise, ¼ cup sour cream and ½ teaspoon curry powder in small bowl. Stir in 2 tablespoons minced fresh cilantro.

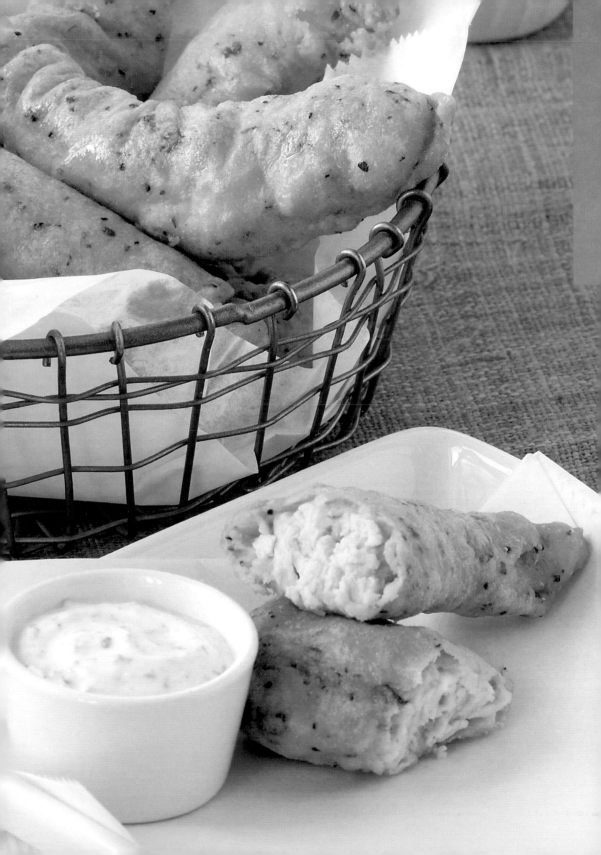

Chicken and Vegetable Risotto

    Olive oil cooking spray

2 cups sliced mushrooms

½ cup chopped onion (about 1 small)

4 cloves garlic, minced

¼ cup finely chopped fresh parsley *or* 1 tablespoon dried parsley flakes

3 tablespoons finely chopped fresh basil *or* 1 tablespoon dried basil

6 cups reduced-sodium chicken broth

1½ cups uncooked arborio rice

2 cups broccoli florets, cooked crisp-tender

1 cup chopped cooked chicken

4 plum tomatoes, chopped

½ teaspoon salt

½ teaspoon black pepper

2 tablespoons grated Parmesan or Romano cheese

1. Spray large nonstick saucepan with cooking spray; heat over medium heat. Add mushrooms, onion and garlic; cook and stir about 5 minutes or until tender. Add parsley and basil; cook and stir 1 minute.

2. Heat broth to a simmer in medium saucepan. Keep warm.

3. Add rice to mushroom mixture; cook and stir over medium heat 1 minute. Add broth, ½ cup at a time, stirring constantly until broth is absorbed before adding next ½ cup. Continue adding broth and stirring until rice is tender and mixture is creamy, 20 to 25 minutes.

4. Add broccoli, chicken, tomatoes, salt and pepper; cook and stir about 3 minutes or until heated through. Sprinkle with cheese.   *Makes 4 servings*

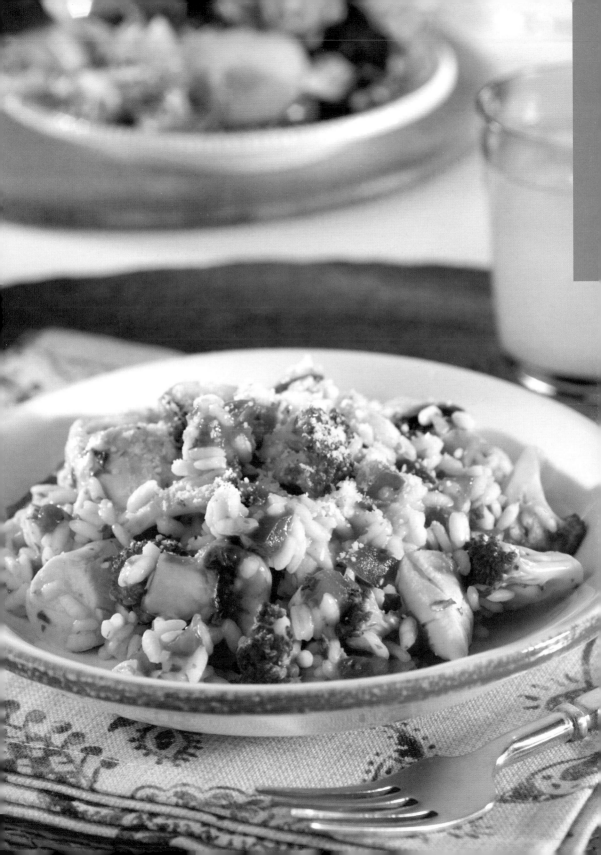

Cornish Hens with Wild Rice and Pine Nut Pilaf

⅓ **cup uncooked wild rice**

4 **Cornish hens (about 1¼ pounds each)**

1 **bunch green onions, cut into 2-inch pieces**

3 **tablespoons olive oil, divided**

3 **tablespoons gluten-free soy sauce**

⅓ **cup pine nuts**

1 **cup chopped onion**

1 **teaspoon dried basil**

2 **cloves garlic, minced**

2 **jalapeño peppers,* seeded and minced**

½ **teaspoon salt**

   Black pepper

*Jalapeño peppers can sting and irritate the skin, so wear rubber gloves when handling peppers and do not touch your eyes.

1. Preheat oven to 425°F. Cook rice according to package directions.

2. Stuff hens equally with green onions; place on rack in roasting pan. Roast 15 minutes. Meanwhile, combine 1 tablespoon oil and soy sauce in small bowl. Baste hens with 1 tablespoon soy sauce mixture; roast 15 minutes or until cooked through (165°F). Baste with remaining soy sauce mixture. Let stand 15 minutes.

3. Meanwhile, heat large skillet over medium-high heat. Add pine nuts; cook 2 minutes or until golden, stirring constantly. Transfer to plate.

4. Add 1 tablespoon oil, onion and basil to same skillet; cook and stir 5 minutes or until browned. Add garlic; cook and stir 15 seconds. Remove from heat. Add rice, pine nuts, jalapeño peppers, remaining 1 tablespoon oil and salt. Season with black pepper; toss gently to blend. Serve hens with rice mixture.

Makes 4 servings

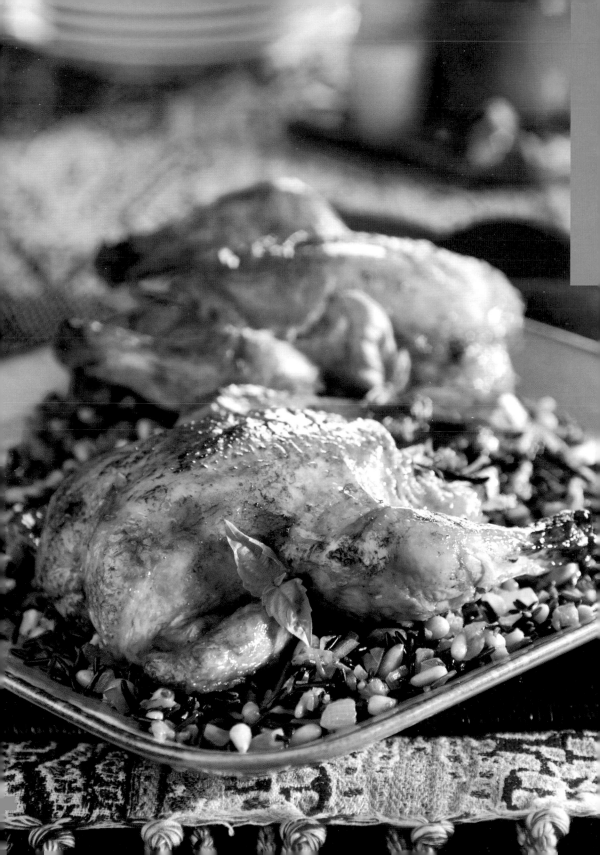

Chipotle Orange BBQ Drumsticks

½ cup gluten-free barbecue sauce
1 to 2 tablespoons minced canned chipotle peppers in adobo sauce
1 teaspoon grated orange peel
8 chicken drumsticks (7 to 8 ounces each), skin removed
1 teaspoon ground cumin

1. Spray grill grid with nonstick cooking spray. Prepare grill for direct cooking.

2. For sauce, combine barbecue sauce, chipotle peppers and orange peel in small bowl. Set aside.

3. Sprinkle drumsticks evenly with cumin.

4. Grill chicken over medium-high heat, covered, 30 to 35 minutes or until cooked through (165°F), turning frequently. Baste with sauce during last 5 minutes, turning and basting until all of sauce is used.

Makes 8 servings

Serving Suggestion: Serve with baked potatoes topped with sour cream and chives.

Tip

It's amazing that gluten can hide in so many prepared food items. While most barbecue sauces are gluten-free, check the labels carefully for any word containing "wheat." Sometimes an ingredient containing wheat gluten (like hydrolyzed wheat protein) will be added to improve the texture of a sauce.

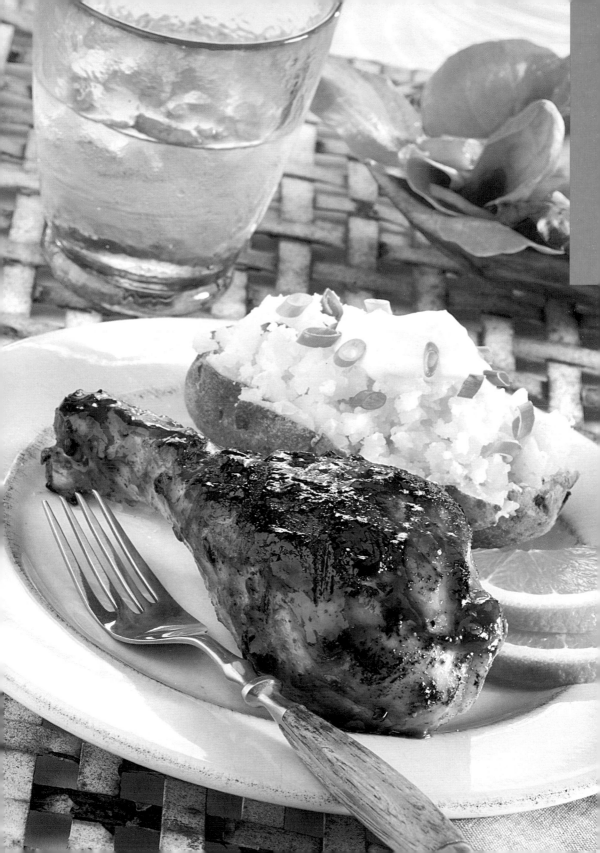

Cajun Chicken and Rice

....

4 chicken drumsticks, skin removed

4 chicken thighs, skin removed

2 teaspoons gluten-free Cajun seasoning

¾ teaspoon salt

2 tablespoons vegetable oil

1 can (about 14 ounces) chicken broth

1 cup uncooked rice

1 medium green bell pepper, coarsely chopped

1 medium red bell pepper, coarsely chopped

½ cup finely chopped green onions

2 cloves garlic, minced

½ teaspoon dried thyme

¼ teaspoon ground turmeric

1. Preheat oven to 350°F. Lightly coat 13×9-inch baking dish with nonstick cooking spray.

2. Sprinkle both sides of chicken with Cajun seasoning and salt. Heat oil in large skillet over medium-high heat. Add chicken; cook 8 to 10 minutes or until browned on all sides. Transfer to plate.

3. Add broth to skillet. Bring to a boil, scraping browned bits from bottom of skillet. Stir in rice, bell peppers, green onions, garlic, thyme and turmeric. Pour into prepared baking dish. Place chicken on top. Cover tightly with foil. Bake 1 hour or until chicken is cooked through (165°F).   *Makes 6 servings*

Variation: For a one-dish meal, use an ovenproof skillet. Place browned chicken on mixture in skillet, then cover and bake as directed.

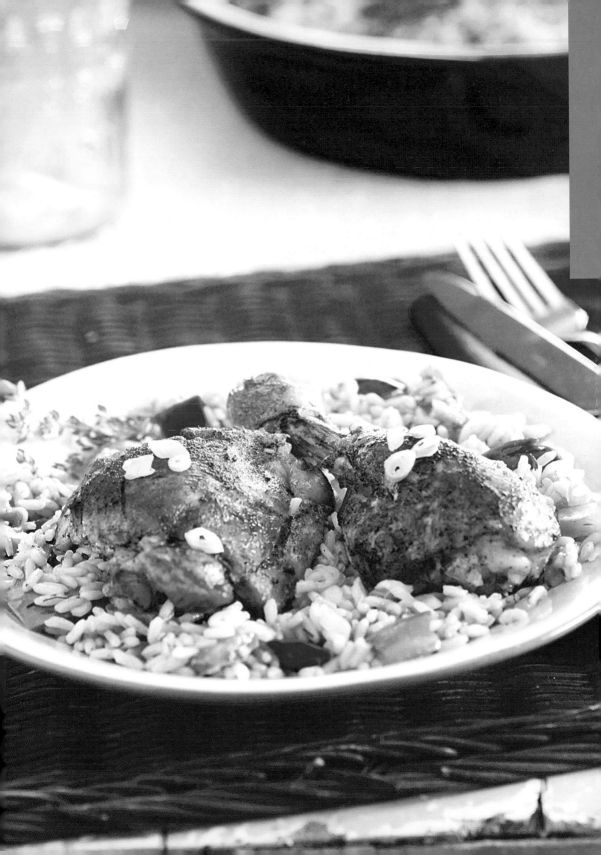

Chicken and Bacon Skewers

¼ **cup lemon juice**
¼ **cup gluten-free soy sauce**
2 **tablespoons packed brown sugar**
1½ **teaspoons lemon pepper**
2 **boneless skinless chicken breasts, cut into 1-inch cubes**
1 **teaspoon coarsely ground black pepper**
½ **pound bacon, cut in half crosswise**
Lemon wedges (optional)

1. Combine lemon juice, soy sauce, brown sugar and lemon pepper in large resealable food storage bag; mix well. Remove ¼ cup marinade; set aside. Add chicken to bag; seal. Marinate in refrigerator at least 30 minutes.

2. Preheat broiler. Sprinkle black pepper over bacon; gently press to adhere. Fold each slice in half. Remove chicken from bag; discard marinade. Alternately thread chicken and bacon onto skewers.

3. Broil skewers 10 to 15 minutes or until chicken is cooked through and bacon is crisp, turning occasionally. Brush several times with reserved marinade. Garnish with lemon wedges. *Makes 2 servings*

Note: If using wooden skewers, soak in water 20 to 30 minutes before using to prevent scorching.

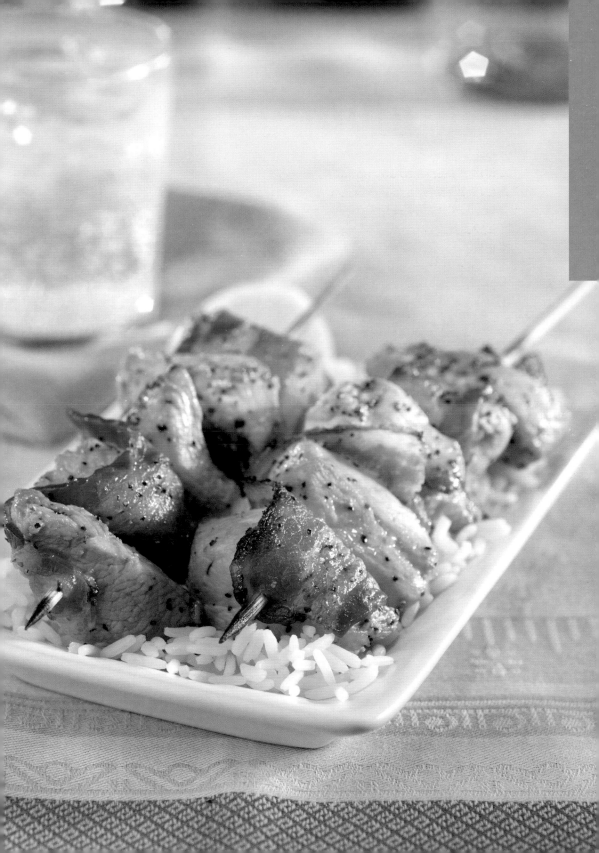

Chicken Saltimbocca

¼ cup coarsely chopped fresh basil

2 tablespoons minced fresh chives

2 teaspoons olive oil

1 clove garlic, minced

½ teaspoon dried oregano

½ teaspoon dried sage

4 boneless skinless chicken breasts (about 4 ounces each)

2 slices (1 ounce each) smoked ham, cut in half

Nonstick cooking spray

½ cup chicken broth

1 cup pasta sauce

2 cups hot cooked spaghetti squash (see Note)

1. Combine basil, chives, oil, garlic, oregano and sage in small bowl. Pound chicken between waxed paper to ½- to ¾-inch thickness with flat side of meat mallet or rolling pin. Spread herb mixture evenly over chicken. Place 1 ham slice over herb mixture; roll up to enclose filling. Secure with toothpicks.

2. Spray medium nonstick skillet with cooking spray; heat over medium-high heat. Cook chicken, seam side up, 2 to 3 minutes or until browned. Turn; cook 2 to 3 minutes or until browned. Add broth; reduce heat to medium-low. Cover and simmer 20 minutes or until cooked through.

3. Remove chicken to cutting board, leaving liquid in skillet. Let chicken stand 5 minutes. Add pasta sauce to same skillet; cook over medium-low heat 2 to 3 minutes or until heated through, stirring occasionally.

4. Remove toothpicks from chicken and cut crosswise into slices. Serve chicken with squash. Top with sauce. *Makes 4 servings*

Note: To cook spaghetti squash, cut squash in half lengthwise; remove and discard seeds. Place, cut side down, in a microwavable baking dish. Add ½ cup water. Cover; cook on HIGH 10 to 15 minutes or until soft. Let cool 15 minutes. Scrape out squash strands with a fork.

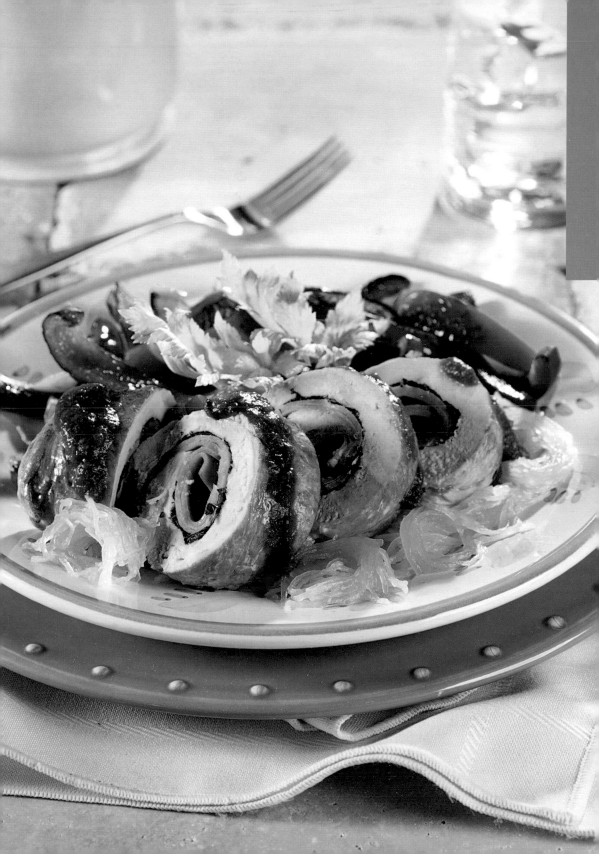

Easy Ethnic

Better-Than-Take-Out Fried Rice

3 tablespoons gluten-free soy sauce

1 tablespoon unseasoned rice vinegar

⅛ teaspoon red pepper flakes

1 red bell pepper

1 tablespoon peanut or vegetable oil

6 green onions, cut into 1-inch pieces

1 tablespoon grated fresh ginger

1½ teaspoons minced garlic

½ pound boneless pork loin or tenderloin, cut into 1-inch pieces

2 cups shredded coleslaw mix

1 package (about 8 ounces) cooked whole grain brown rice

1. Combine soy sauce, vinegar and red pepper flakes in small bowl.

2. Cut bell pepper into 1-inch pieces or cut into decorative shapes using small cookie cutters.

3. Heat oil in large nonstick skillet or wok over medium-high heat. Add bell pepper, green onions, ginger and garlic; stir-fry 1 minute. Add pork; stir-fry 2 to 3 minutes or until pork is cooked through.

4. Stir in coleslaw mix, rice and soy sauce mixture; cook and stir 1 minute or until heated through.   *Makes 4 servings*

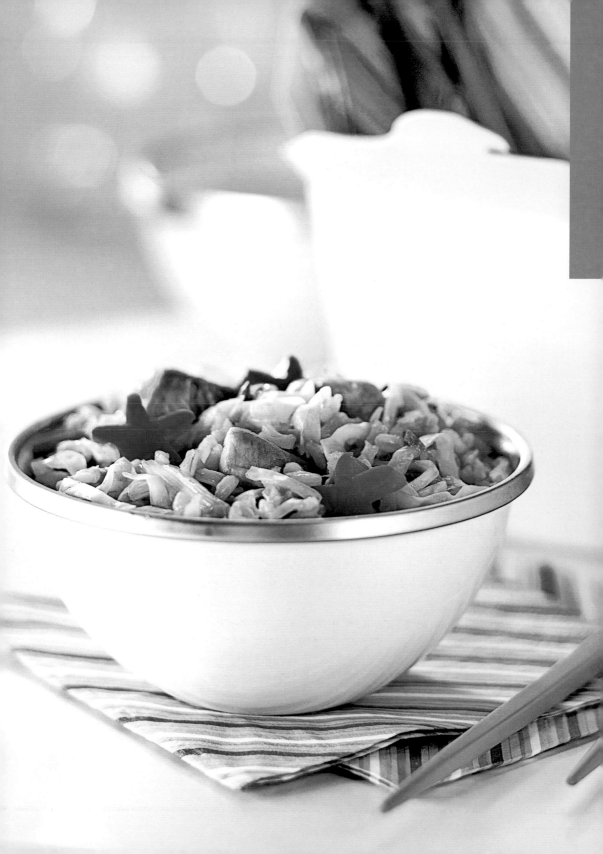

Sweet Potato Gnocchi

1½ pounds sweet potatoes (2 or 3 medium)
¼ cup sweet rice flour,* plus additional for rolling
1 tablespoon lemon juice
1 teaspoon salt
½ teaspoon xanthan gum
½ teaspoon ground nutmeg
½ teaspoon black pepper
¼ teaspoon sugar
2 to 4 tablespoons extra virgin olive oil, divided
1 pound spinach, stemmed

*Sweet rice flour is sometimes labeled mochiko (the Japanese term). It is available in the Asian section of large supermarkets, at Asian grocers and on the Internet.

1. Preheat oven to 375°F. Poke sweet potatoes with fork in several places. Bake 50 to 60 minutes or until very soft. Remove and discard skins. Press potatoes through ricer or mash very well; discard stringy pieces. You should have about 2½ cups mashed sweet potato.

2. Combine sweet potato, rice flour, lemon juice, salt, xanthan gum, nutmeg, pepper and sugar in medium bowl. Mix well.

3. Line baking sheet with foil. Heavily flour cutting board or work surface. Working in batches, scoop portions of dough onto cutting board and roll into ½-inch-thick rope using floured hands. Cut into ¾-inch pieces. Shape each piece into oval; make ridges with tines of fork. Transfer to prepared baking sheet. Freeze gnocchi on baking sheet at least 30 minutes.*

4. Heat 1 tablespoon oil in large nonstick skillet. Add frozen gnocchi in batches and cook, turning once, until lightly browned and warmed through, adding additional oil as needed to prevent sticking. Remove from skillet and keep warm.

5. Add remaining oil to coat bottom of skillet. Add spinach; cook and stir 30 seconds or just until barely wilted. Serve gnocchi with spinach.

Makes 4 servings

*Gnocchi may be made ahead to this point and frozen for up to 24 hours. For longer storage, transfer frozen gnocchi to covered freezer container.

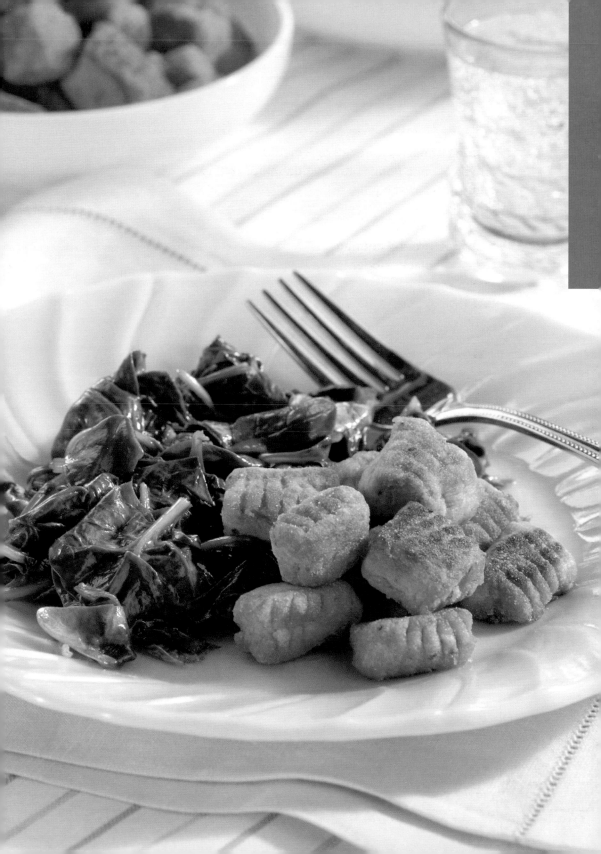

Midweek Moussaka

1 eggplant (about 1 pound), cut into ¼-inch slices
2 tablespoons olive oil
1 pound ground beef
1 can (about 14 ounces) stewed tomatoes, drained
¼ cup red wine
2 tablespoons tomato paste
2 teaspoons sugar
¾ teaspoon salt
½ teaspoon dried oregano
¼ teaspoon ground cinnamon
¼ teaspoon black pepper
⅛ teaspoon ground allspice
4 ounces cream cheese
¼ cup milk
¼ cup grated Parmesan cheese

1. Preheat broiler. Coat 8-inch square baking dish with nonstick cooking spray.

2. Line baking sheet with foil. Arrange eggplant slices on foil, overlapping slightly if necessary. Brush with oil; broil 5 to 6 inches from heat 4 minutes on each side. *Reduce oven temperature to 350°F.*

3. Meanwhile, brown beef in large nonstick skillet over medium-high heat 6 to 8 minutes, stirring to break up meat. Drain fat. Add tomatoes, wine, tomato paste, sugar, salt, oregano, cinnamon, pepper and allspice. Bring to a boil, breaking up large pieces of tomato with spoon. Reduce heat to medium-low; cover and simmer 10 minutes.

4. Place cream cheese and milk in small microwavable bowl. Cover and microwave on HIGH 1 minute. Stir with fork until smooth.

5. Arrange half of eggplant slices in prepared baking dish. Spoon half of meat sauce over eggplant; sprinkle with half of Parmesan cheese. Repeat layers. Spoon cream cheese mixture evenly over top. Bake 20 minutes or until heated through. Sprinkle lightly with additional cinnamon, if desired. Let stand 10 minutes before serving. *Makes 4 servings*

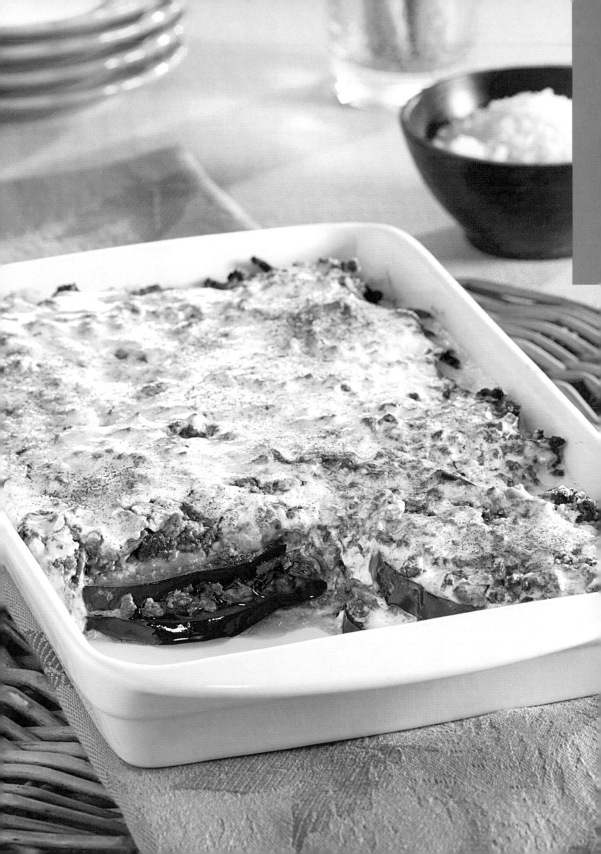

Fiesta Beef Enchiladas

6 ounces ground beef
¼ cup sliced green onions
1 teaspoon minced garlic
1 cup (4 ounces) shredded Mexican cheese blend, divided
1 cup chopped tomato, divided
½ cup corn
½ cup cooked rice
½ cup cooked black beans
¼ cup salsa or picante sauce
6 (6-inch) corn tortillas
½ cup gluten-free enchilada sauce
Chopped lettuce

1. Preheat oven to 375°F. Spray two 20×12-inch sheets of heavy-duty foil with nonstick cooking spray.

2. Brown ground beef in large nonstick skillet over medium-high heat, stirring to break up meat. Drain fat. Add green onions and garlic; cook and stir 2 minutes.

3. Combine meat mixture, ¾ cup cheese, ½ cup tomato, corn, rice, beans and salsa; mix well. Spoon mixture down center of tortillas. Roll up; place 3 enchiladas, seam side down, on each foil sheet. Top with enchilada sauce.

4. Seal packets, leaving head space for heat circulation. Place on baking sheet. Bake 15 minutes.

5. Remove from oven; open packets. Sprinkle with remaining ¼ cup cheese. Reseal packets. Bake 10 minutes or until cheese melts. Serve with lettuce and remaining ½ cup tomato. *Makes 2 servings*

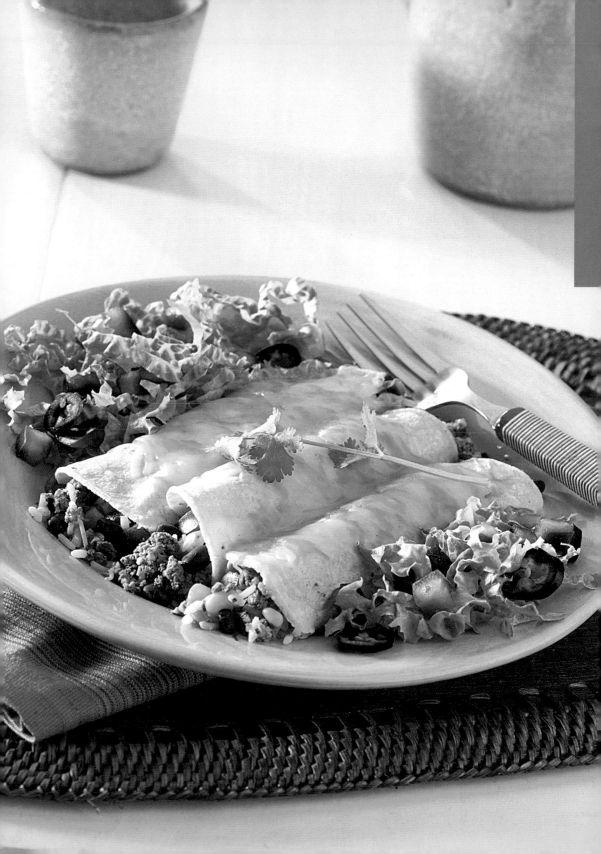

Cellophane Noodles with Minced Pork

32 dried shiitake mushrooms
1 package (about 4 ounces) cellophane noodles*
2 tablespoons minced fresh ginger
2 tablespoons gluten-free black bean sauce
1½ cups chicken broth
1 tablespoon dry sherry
1 tablespoon gluten-free soy sauce
2 tablespoons vegetable oil
6 ounces lean ground pork
3 green onions, sliced
1 jalapeño or other hot pepper, finely chopped**
Cilantro sprigs and hot red peppers (optional)

Cellophane noodles (also called bean threads or glass noodles) are thin, translucent noodles sold in tangled bunches.

**Jalapeño peppers can sting and irritate the skin, so wear rubber gloves when handling peppers and do not touch your eyes.*

1. Place mushrooms in medium bowl; cover with hot water. Let soak 30 minutes or until softened. Squeeze out excess water. Discard stems; cut caps into thin slices.

2. Place noodles in medium bowl; cover with hot water. Let soak 15 minutes or until softened. Drain; cut into 4-inch pieces.

3. Combine ginger and black bean sauce in small bowl. Combine broth, sherry and soy sauce in medium bowl.

4. Heat oil in wok or large skillet over high heat. Add pork; stir-fry about 2 minutes or until no longer pink. Add green onions, jalapeño and black bean sauce mixture; stir-fry 1 minute.

5. Add broth mixture, mushrooms and noodles. Simmer, uncovered, about 5 minutes or until most of liquid is absorbed. Garnish with cilantro and red peppers. *Makes 4 servings*

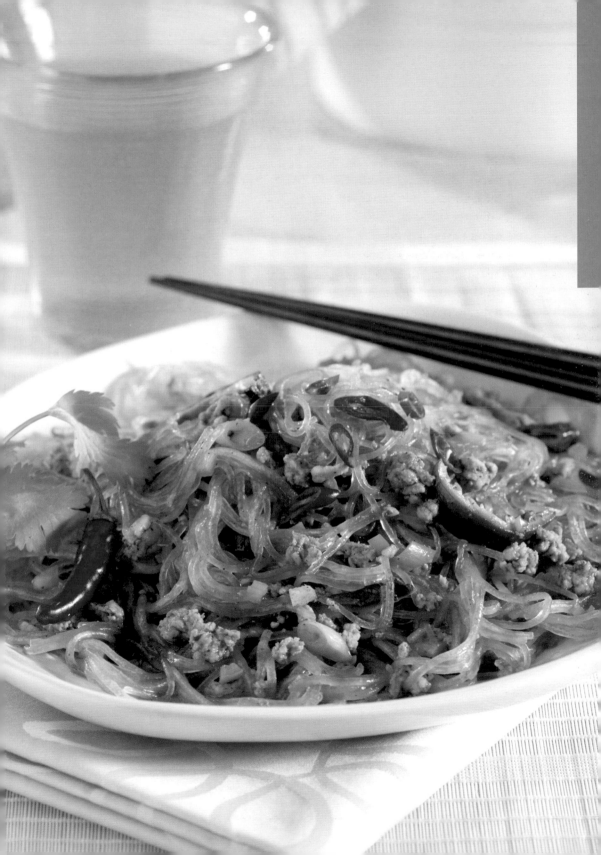

Italian Vegetarian Grill

1 large bell pepper, quartered

1 medium zucchini, cut into ½-inch-thick pieces

½ pound asparagus (about 10 spears)

1 large red onion, cut into ½-inch-thick rounds

¼ cup olive oil

1 teaspoon salt, divided

½ teaspoon Italian seasoning

½ teaspoon black pepper, divided

4 cups water

1 cup uncooked polenta

4 ounces crumbled goat cheese

1. Arrange bell pepper, zucchini and asparagus in single layer on baking sheet. To hold onion together securely, pierce slices horizontally with metal skewers. Add to baking sheet. Combine oil, ½ teaspoon salt, Italian seasoning and ¼ teaspoon black pepper in small bowl. Brush mixture generously over vegetables, turning to coat all sides.

2. Prepare grill for direct cooking. Meanwhile, bring water to a boil with remaining ½ teaspoon salt in large saucepan. Gradually whisk in polenta. Reduce heat to medium. Cook, stirring constantly, until polenta thickens and begins to pull away from side of pan. Stir in remaining ¼ teaspoon black pepper. Keep warm.

3. Grill vegetables over medium-high heat, covered, 10 to 15 minutes or until tender, turning once. Place bell pepper in large bowl. Cover; let stand 5 minutes to loosen skin. When cool enough to handle, peel off charred skin. Cut all vegetables into bite-size pieces.

4. Serve polenta topped with vegetables; sprinkle with goat cheese.

Makes 4 servings

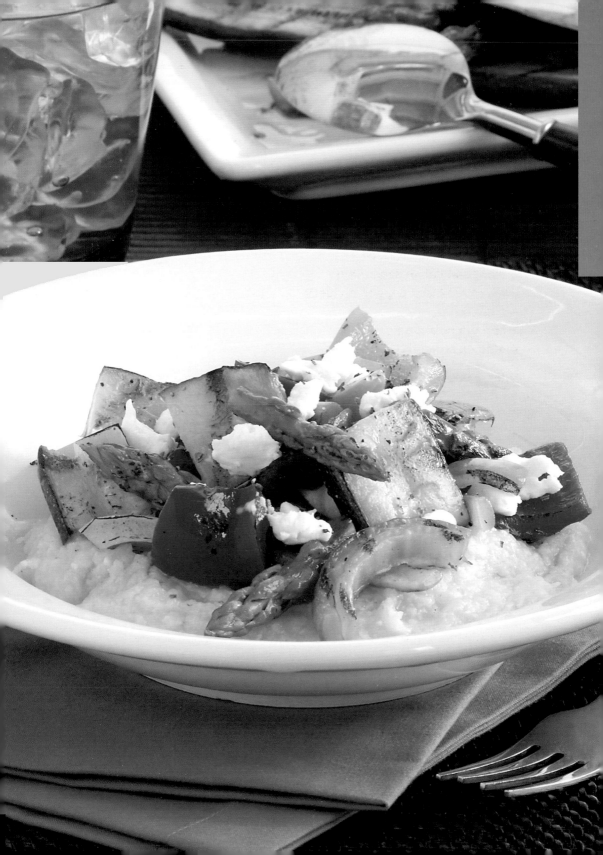

Cheese Blintzes

1 cup rice flour
¼ teaspoon salt
¼ teaspoon ground nutmeg
1 cup half-and-half
3 tablespoons butter, melted, divided
1½ teaspoons vanilla, divided
3 eggs
1 container (15 ounces) ricotta cheese
2 tablespoons powdered sugar
Preserves, applesauce or sour cream

1. Combine rice flour, salt and nutmeg in medium bowl. Gradually whisk in half-and-half until smooth.

2. Add 2 tablespoons butter and ½ teaspoon vanilla. Whisk in eggs, one at a time, until batter is smooth with consistency of heavy cream.

3. Heat 8- or 9-inch nonstick skillet over medium heat. Brush lightly with some of remaining butter. Pour about ¼ cup batter into center of pan. Immediately swirl pan to coat with batter. Cook about 1 minute or until crêpe is dull on top and edges are dry. Turn and cook 30 seconds. Remove to plate; keep warm. Repeat with remaining batter.

4. Meanwhile, combine ricotta, powdered sugar and remaining 1 teaspoon vanilla in medium bowl. Fill crêpes with ricotta mixture. Serve with preserves, applesauce or sour cream. *Makes about 14 blintzes*

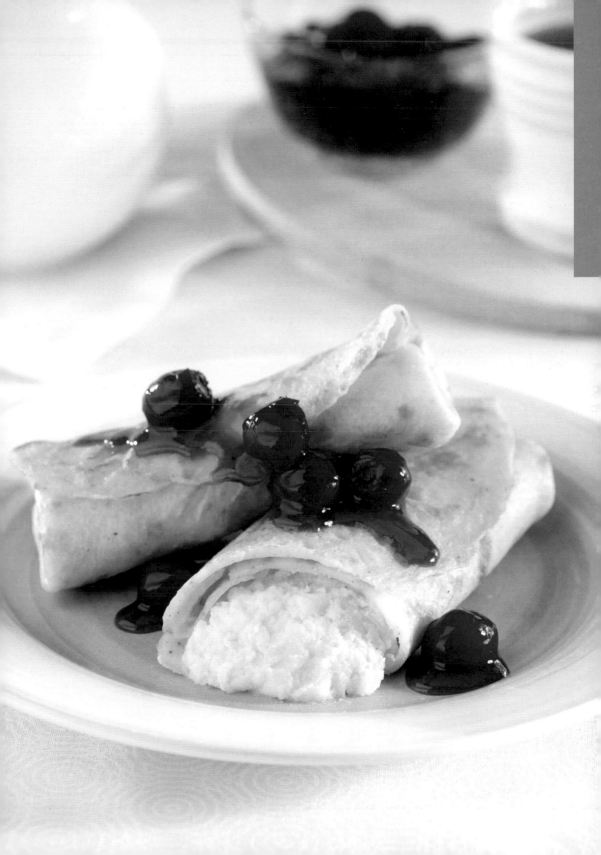

Basil Chicken with Rice Noodles

1 pound boneless skinless chicken breasts, cut into bite-size pieces
5 tablespoons gluten-free soy sauce, divided
1 tablespoon white wine or rice wine
3 cloves garlic, minced
1 tablespoon grated fresh ginger
8 ounces (about half a package) rice noodles
1 red onion, sliced
1 yellow or red bell pepper, cut into strips
2 medium carrots, cut into matchstick-size pieces
2 jalapeño or serrano peppers,* chopped
  Juice of 2 limes
2 tablespoons packed brown sugar
1 to 2 tablespoons vegetable oil
1½ cups loosely packed basil leaves, shredded

*Jalapeño peppers can sting and irritate the skin, so wear rubber gloves when handling peppers and do not touch your eyes.

1. Place chicken in shallow dish. Combine 3 tablespoons soy sauce, wine, garlic and ginger in small bowl. Pour over chicken and stir to coat. Marinate at room temperature 30 minutes or refrigerate up to 2 hours.

2. Place noodles in medium bowl. Cover with hot water; let stand 15 minutes or until soft. Drain well.

3. Combine onion, bell pepper, carrots and jalapeño peppers in medium bowl. For sauce, stir remaining 2 tablespoons soy sauce, lime juice and brown sugar in small bowl.

4. Heat large skillet or wok over medium-high heat. Add oil to coat. Add chicken with marinade; cook and stir until no longer pink. Add vegetables; stir-fry 4 to 6 minutes or until vegetables begin to soften.

5. Stir sauce to dissolve sugar and add to skillet. Cook and stir 2 minutes. Stir in noodles and basil. *Makes 4 to 6 servings*

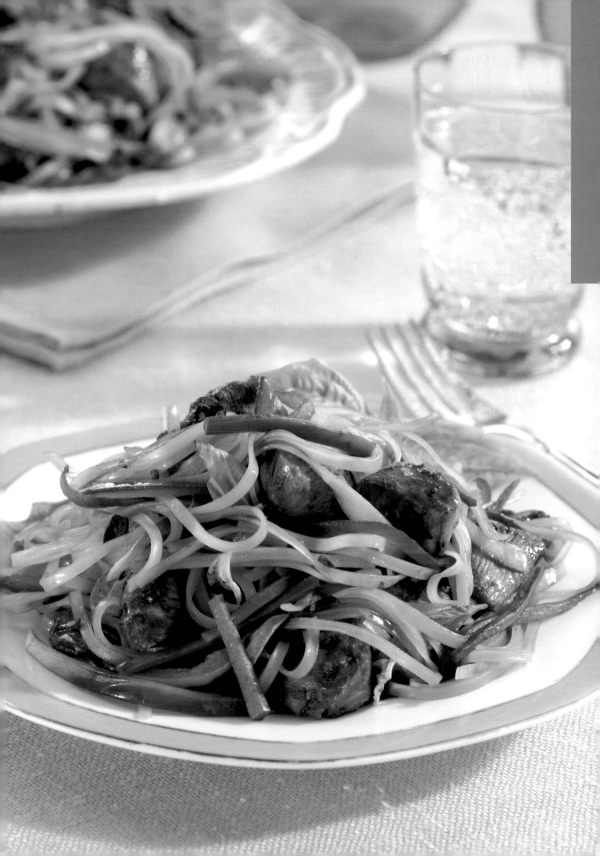

Indian-Inspired Chicken with Raita

1 cup plain yogurt

2 cloves garlic, minced

1 teaspoon salt

1 teaspoon ground coriander

1 teaspoon ground ginger

½ teaspoon ground turmeric

½ teaspoon ground cinnamon

½ teaspoon ground cumin

¼ teaspoon ground red pepper

1 (5- to 6-pound) chicken, cut into 8 pieces (about 4 pounds chicken parts)

Raita

2 medium cucumbers (about 1 pound), peeled, seeded and thinly sliced

⅓ cup plain yogurt

2 tablespoons chopped fresh cilantro

1 clove garlic, minced

¼ teaspoon salt

⅛ teaspoon black pepper

1. Mix yogurt, garlic, salt, coriander, ginger, turmeric, cinnamon, cumin and red pepper in medium bowl. Place chicken in large resealable food storage bag. Add yogurt mixture; marinate in refrigerator 4 to 24 hours, turning occasionally.

2. Preheat broiler. Cover baking sheet with foil. Place chicken on prepared baking sheet. Broil 6 inches from heat about 30 minutes or until cooked through (165°F), turning once.

3. Meanwhile, prepare Raita. Mix cucumbers, yogurt, cilantro, garlic, salt and black pepper in small bowl. Serve with chicken.   *Makes 6 to 8 servings*

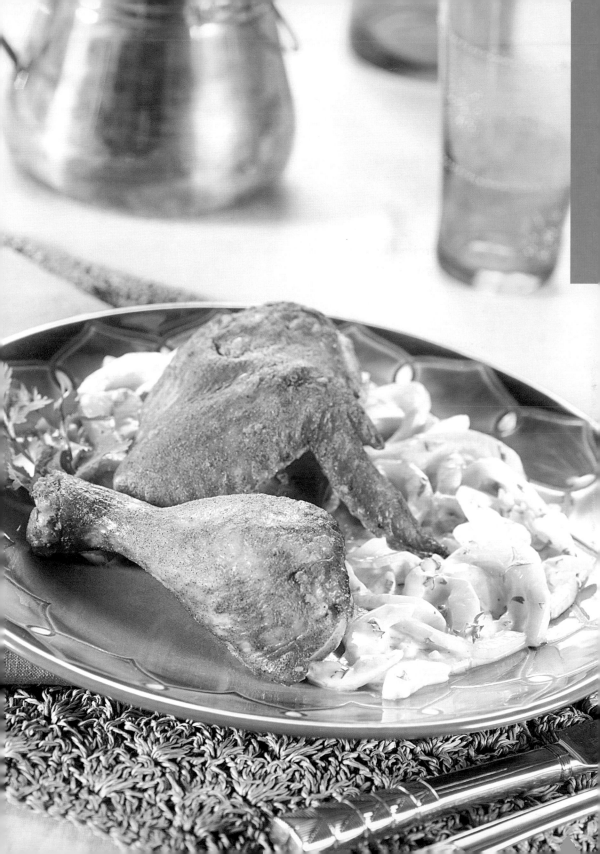

Glazed Tofu with Rice

1 package (14 ounces) extra firm tofu
1 cup gluten-free stir-fry sauce, divided
1 cup uncooked long grain rice
4 medium carrots, chopped (about 1 cup)
4 ounces snow peas, halved (about 1 cup)

1. Slice tofu in half crosswise. Cut each half into 2 triangles. Place tofu triangles on cutting board between layers of paper towels. Place another cutting board on top to press moisture out of tofu. Let stand about 15 minutes.

2. Spread ½ cup stir-fry sauce in baking dish. Place tofu in sauce; marinate at room temperature 30 minutes, turning after 15 minutes.

3. Meanwhile, cook rice according to package directions. Keep warm.

4. Spray grill pan with nonstick cooking spray; heat over medium-high heat. Place tofu in pan; grill 6 to 8 minutes or until lightly browned, turning after 4 minutes.

5. Meanwhile, pour remaining ½ cup stir-fry sauce into large nonstick skillet; heat over medium-high heat. Add carrots and snow peas; cook and stir 4 to 6 minutes or until crisp-tender. Add rice; stir to combine.

6. Serve tofu on rice mixture. *Makes 4 servings*

Tip

Prepared stir-fry sauce comes in many varieties and they all include soy sauce, so it's extremely important to check labels for gluten. If you have trouble finding a safe prepared sauce, just make your own. Combine gluten-free soy sauce with some minced garlic and ginger. Add a bit of brown sugar and heat things up with some red pepper if you like. Sesame seed or sesame oil is also a nice addition.

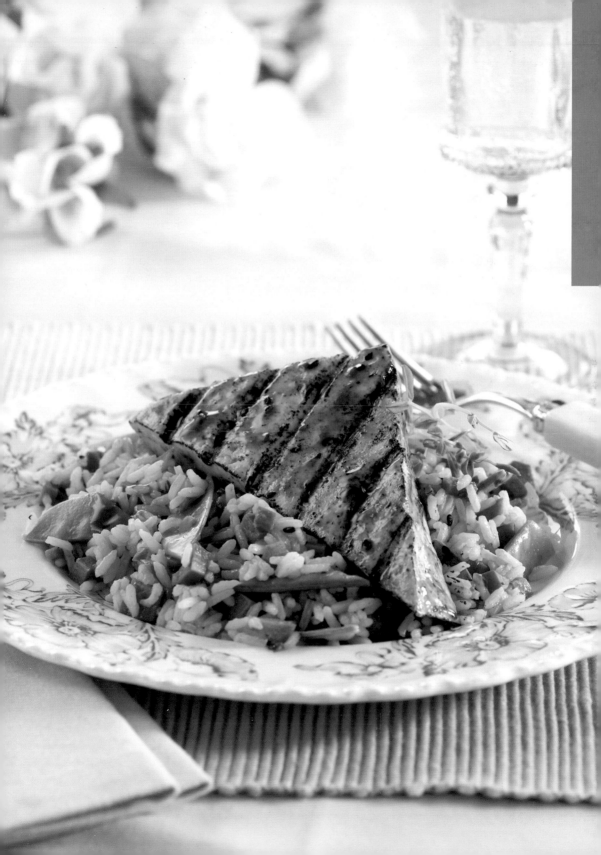

Light Bites

Spanish Tortilla

1 teaspoon olive oil

1 cup thinly sliced peeled potato

1 small zucchini, thinly sliced

¼ cup chopped onion

1 clove garlic, minced

1 cup shredded cooked chicken

8 eggs

½ teaspoon salt

½ teaspoon black pepper

¼ teaspoon red pepper flakes

Fresh tomato salsa (optional)

1. Heat oil in 10-inch nonstick skillet over medium-high heat. Add potato, zucchini, onion and garlic; cook and stir about 5 minutes or until potato is tender, turning frequently. Stir in chicken; cook 1 minute.

2. Meanwhile, whisk eggs, salt, black pepper and red pepper flakes in large bowl. Carefully pour egg mixture into skillet. Reduce heat to low. Cover and cook 12 to 15 minutes or until egg mixture is set in center.

3. Loosen edges of tortilla and slide onto large serving platter. Let stand 5 minutes before cutting into wedges. Serve warm or at room temperature. Serve with salsa, if desired. *Makes 10 to 12 servings*

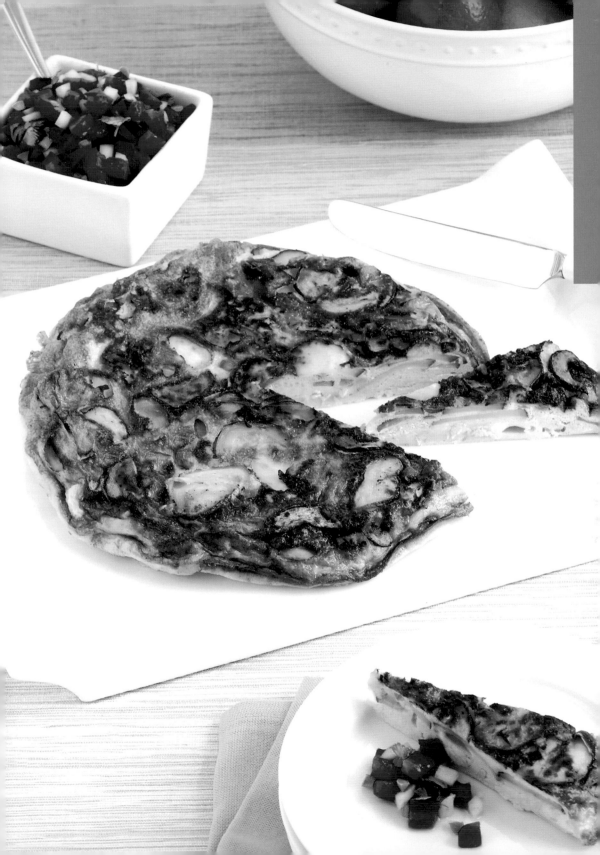

Winter Squash Risotto

2 tablespoons olive oil
1 small butternut or medium delicata squash, peeled and
     cut into 1-inch pieces (2 cups)
1 large shallot or small onion, finely chopped
½ teaspoon paprika
¼ teaspoon dried thyme
¼ teaspoon salt
¼ teaspoon black pepper
 1 cup uncooked arborio rice
¼ cup dry white wine (optional)
 4 to 5 cups hot gluten-free vegetable broth
½ cup grated Parmesan or Romano cheese

1. Heat oil in large skillet over medium heat. Add squash; cook and stir 3 minutes. Add shallot; cook and stir 3 to 4 minutes or until squash is almost tender. Stir in paprika, thyme, salt and pepper. Add rice; stir to coat.

2. Add wine, if desired; cook and stir until wine evaporates. Add broth, ½ cup at a time, stirring constantly until broth is absorbed before adding next ½ cup. Continue adding broth and stirring until rice is tender and consistency is creamy. (Total cooking time will be 20 to 30 minutes.)

3. Sprinkle with cheese just before serving. *Makes 4 to 6 servings*

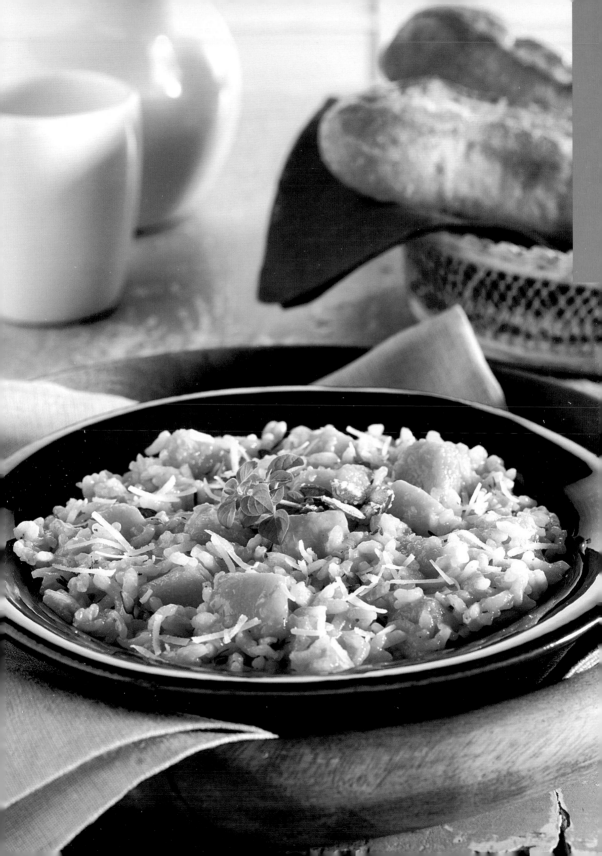

Mini Carnitas Tacos

1½ pounds boneless pork loin, cut into 1-inch cubes
1 onion, finely chopped
½ cup reduced-sodium chicken broth
1 tablespoon chili powder
2 teaspoons ground cumin
1 teaspoon dried oregano
½ teaspoon minced canned chipotle peppers in adobo sauce (optional)
½ cup pico de gallo or salsa
2 tablespoons chopped fresh cilantro
½ teaspoon salt
12 (6-inch) corn tortillas
¾ cup (3 ounces) shredded sharp Cheddar cheese
3 tablespoons sour cream

Slow Cooker Directions

1. Combine pork, onion, broth, chili powder, cumin, oregano and chipotle, if desired, in slow cooker. Cover; cook on LOW 6 hours or on HIGH 3 hours or until pork is very tender. Pour off excess cooking liquid.

2. Shred pork with two forks; stir in pico de gallo, cilantro and salt. Cover and keep warm.

3. Cut 3 circles from each tortilla with 2-inch biscuit cutter. Top with pork, cheese and sour cream. *Makes 12 servings (36 mini tacos)*

Tip

Carnitas means "little meats" in Spanish. This dish is usually made with an inexpensive cut of pork that is simmered for a long time until it falls to pieces. The meat is then browned in pork fat. The slow cooker makes the long, slow cooking process easy to manage and skipping the final browning lowers the fat content.

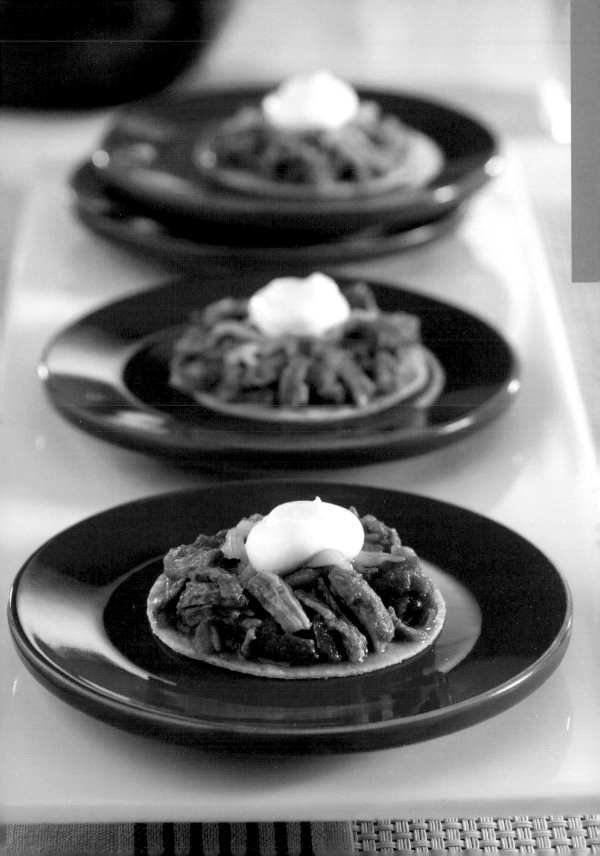

Crustless Ham & Spinach Tart

- 1 teaspoon olive oil
- 1 cup finely chopped onion
- 2 cloves garlic, minced
- 1 package (10 ounces) frozen chopped spinach, thawed and squeezed dry
- 3 slices deli ham, cut into strips (3 ounces total)
- 1 cup milk
- 3 eggs
- ¼ cup plus 2 tablespoons grated Parmesan cheese, divided
- 1 tablespoon minced fresh basil *or* 2 teaspoons dried basil
- ½ teaspoon black pepper
- ⅛ teaspoon ground nutmeg

1. Preheat oven to 350°F. Lightly spray 9-inch glass pie plate with nonstick cooking spray.

2. Heat oil in medium nonstick skillet over medium-high heat. Add onion and cook 2 minutes or until soft, stirring occasionally. Add garlic and cook 1 minute. Stir in spinach and ham. Spread evenly in prepared pie plate.

3. Combine milk, eggs, ¼ cup cheese, basil, pepper and nutmeg in medium bowl. Pour over spinach mixture. Bake 50 minutes or until knife inserted into center comes out clean. Sprinkle with remaining 2 tablespoons cheese.

Makes 6 servings

Tip

This easy recipe is perfect for breakfast, brunch, lunch or a light dinner. You'll never miss the crust and the ingredients can be customized to suit your taste and what you have on hand. Crumbled bacon and asparagus would be good substitutes for the ham and spinach.

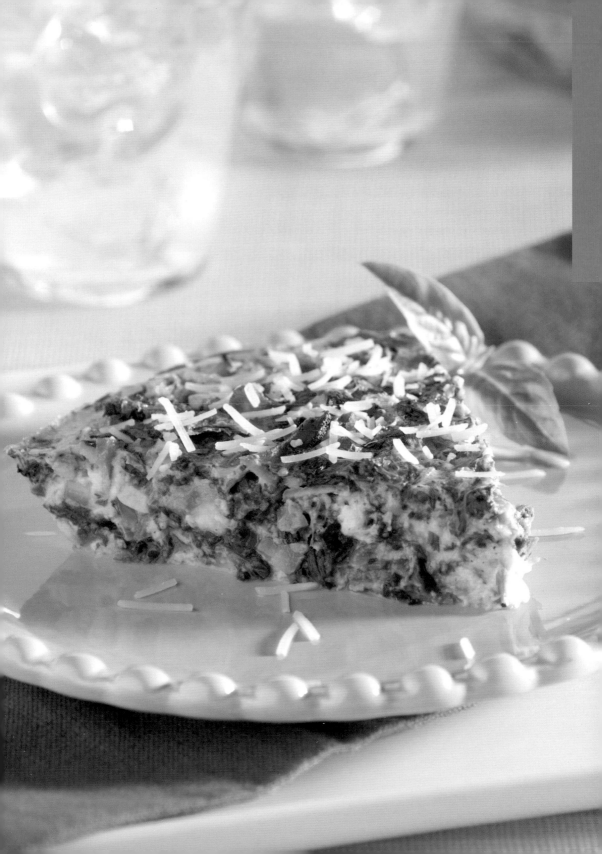

Apple Pancakes

     2 tablespoons plus 2 teaspoons dairy-free stick margarine
  1¼ cups soymilk or other milk
     2 eggs, beaten
  1¼ cups Gluten-Free All-Purpose Flour Blend (recipe follows)*
     ¼ cup finely chopped dried apple
     ¼ cup golden raisins
     3 tablespoons sugar
     1 tablespoon baking powder
     1 teaspoon ground cinnamon
     ½ teaspoon salt
        Maple syrup and additional dairy-free margarine
*Or use any all-purpose gluten-free flour blend that does not contain xanthan gum.

1. Melt margarine in large skillet or griddle over medium heat. Pour into medium bowl, leaving thin film of margarine on skillet. Whisk soymilk and eggs into margarine in bowl.

2. Combine flour blend, apple, raisins, sugar, baking powder, cinnamon and salt in large bowl. Add soymilk mixture; stir to combine.

3. Pour ¼ cup batter into skillet for each pancake. Cook over medium heat 2 to 3 minutes on each side or until golden. Serve with maple syrup and additional margarine.   *Makes 10 to 12 pancakes*

Gluten-Free All-Purpose Flour Blend: Combine 1 cup white rice flour, 1 cup sorghum flour, 1 cup tapioca flour, 1 cup cornstarch and 1 cup almond or coconut flour in large bowl. Whisk to make sure flours are evenly distributed. The recipe can be doubled or tripled. Store in airtight container in the refrigerator. Makes about 5 cups.

Variation: Substitute ¼ cup chopped pecans for the raisins.

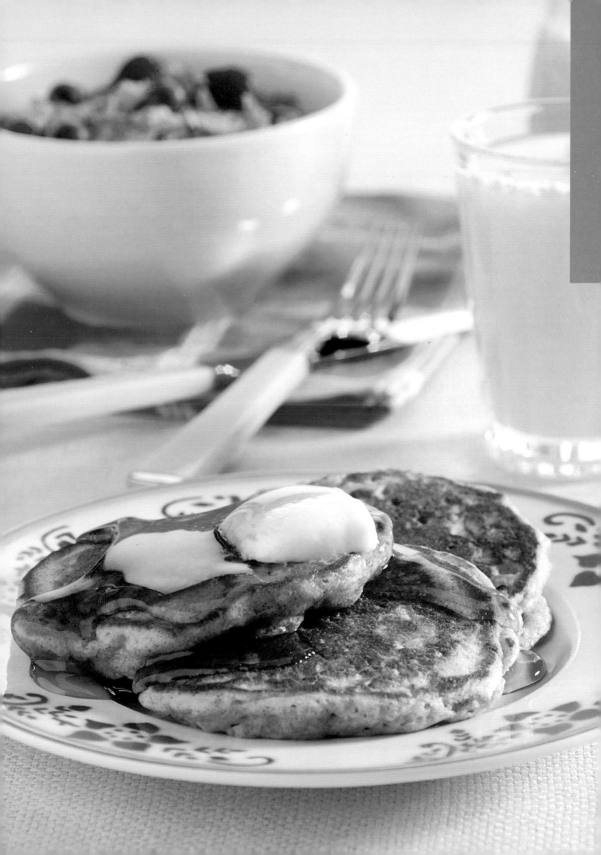

Asiago and Asparagus Risotto-Style Rice

2 cups chopped onions
1 cup uncooked converted rice
2 cloves garlic, minced
1 can (about 14 ounces) gluten-free vegetable broth
½ pound asparagus spears, trimmed and cut into 1-inch pieces
1 cup half-and-half, divided
½ cup (about 4 ounces) shredded Asiago cheese, plus additional
 for garnish
¼ cup (½ stick) butter, cut into small pieces
2 ounces pine nuts or slivered almonds, toasted
1 teaspoon salt

Slow Cooker Directions

1. Combine onions, rice, garlic and broth in slow cooker; stir until well blended. Cover; cook on HIGH 2 hours or until rice is done.

2. Stir in asparagus and ½ cup half-and-half. Cover; cook 20 to 30 minutes or until asparagus is crisp-tender.

3. Stir in remaining ½ cup half-and-half, ½ cup cheese, butter, nuts and salt. Cover and let stand 5 minutes to allow cheese to melt slightly. Fluff with fork and garnish with additional cheese. *Makes 4 servings*

Tip

Risotto is a classic creamy rice dish of northern Italy. It can be made with a wide variety of ingredients; fresh vegetables and cheeses such as Asiago work especially well in risottos. Parmesan cheese, shellfish, white wine and herbs are also popular additions.

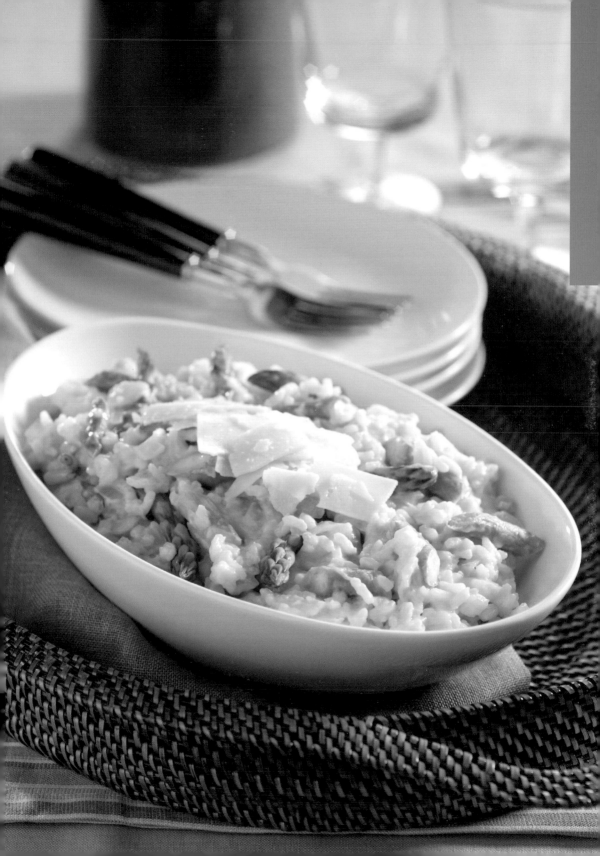

Apple-Stuffed Acorn Squash

¼ **cup raisins**
2 **acorn squash (about 4 inches in diameter)**
Butter-flavored cooking spray
2 **tablespoons sugar**
¼ **teaspoon ground cinnamon**
2 **medium Fuji apples**
2 **tablespoons butter**

1. Cover raisins with warm water and soak 20 minutes. Preheat oven to 375°F.

2. Cut squash into quarters; remove seeds. Spray squash with cooking spray; place on baking sheet. Combine sugar and cinnamon in small bowl; sprinkle squash with half of cinnamon mixture. Bake 10 minutes.

3. Meanwhile, cut apples into quarters; remove cores. Chop apples into ½-inch pieces. Drain raisins. Melt butter in medium saucepan over medium heat. Add apples, raisins and remaining cinnamon mixture; cook and stir 1 minute. Top partially baked squash with apple mixture. Bake 30 to 35 minutes or until apples and squash are tender.   *Makes 8 servings*

Bacon-Wrapped BBQ Chicken

8 **chicken tenders (about 1 pound)**
½ **teaspoon paprika or ground cumin**
8 **slices bacon**
½ **cup gluten-free barbecue sauce, divided**

1. Preheat broiler. Line broiler pan with foil.

2. Sprinkle chicken tenders with paprika. Wrap each chicken tender with slice of bacon in spiral pattern; place on prepared pan.

3. Broil chicken 4 minutes. Turn and broil 2 minutes. Brush with ¼ cup barbecue sauce; broil 2 minutes. Turn and brush with remaining ¼ cup barbecue sauce; broil 2 minutes or until chicken is no longer pink in center.

Makes 4 servings

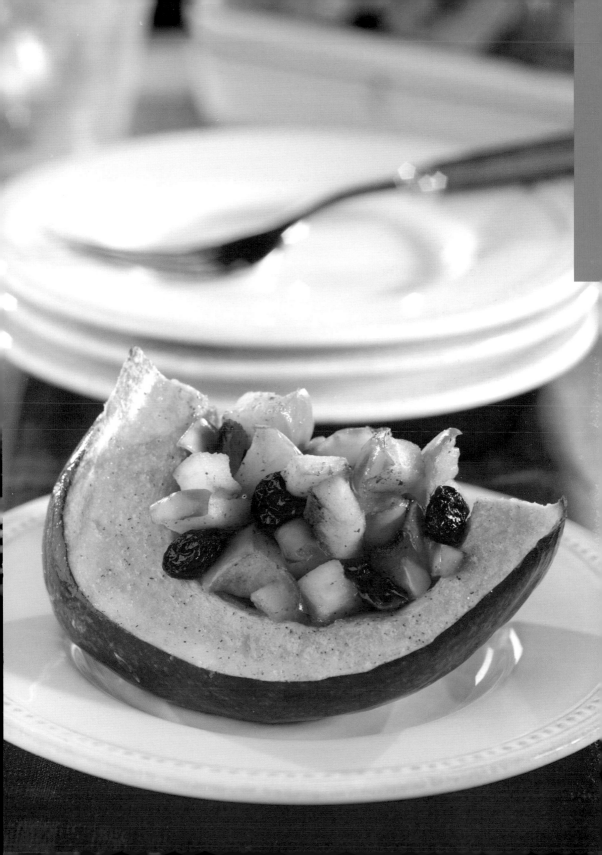

Cheesy Quichettes

12 slices bacon, crisp-cooked and crumbled
6 eggs, beaten
¼ cup whole milk
1½ cups refrigerated shredded hash brown potatoes
¼ cup chopped fresh parsley
½ teaspoon salt
1½ cups (6 ounces) shredded Mexican cheese blend with jalapeño peppers

1. Preheat oven to 400°F. Lightly spray 12 standard (2½-inch) muffin cups with nonstick cooking spray.

2. Place equal amounts of bacon into prepared muffin cups. Beat eggs and milk in medium bowl. Add potatoes, parsley and salt; mix well. Spoon mixture evenly into muffin cups.

3. Bake 15 minutes or until knife inserted into centers comes out almost clean. Sprinkle with cheese; let stand 3 minutes or until cheese melts. (Egg mixture will continue to cook while standing.*) To remove from pan, gently run knife around outer edges and lift out with fork.   *Makes 12 quichettes*
Standing also allows for easier removal of quichettes from pan.

Tip

Going gluten-free means becoming a label detective. Fortunately, by law any ingredient or product that contains any form of wheat must list wheat on the label. You will probably encounter some multisyllabic words that sound like they came from a chemistry lab. You'll need to check a list of safe and unsafe ingredients to figure those out. See www.celiac.com for information.

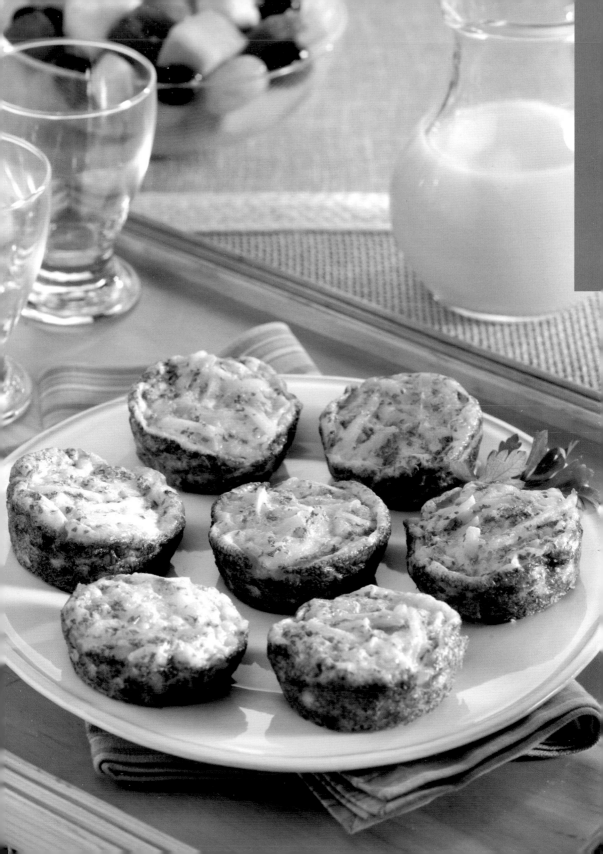

Spring Vegetable Ragoût

1 tablespoon olive oil

2 leeks, thinly sliced

3 cloves garlic, minced

1 package (10 ounces) frozen corn

1 cup gluten-free vegetable broth

½ pound yellow squash, halved lengthwise and cut into ½-inch pieces (about 1¼ cups)

1 package (6 ounces) frozen edamame (soybeans), shelled

4 ounces shredded carrots

3 cups small cherry tomatoes, halved

1 teaspoon dried tarragon

1 teaspoon dried basil

1 teaspoon dried oregano

Salt and black pepper

Minced fresh parsley (optional)

1. Heat oil in large skillet over medium heat. Add leeks and garlic; cook and stir just until fragrant. Add corn, broth, squash, edamame and carrots; cook and stir until squash is tender.

2. Stir in tomatoes, tarragon, basil and oregano. Reduce heat to low. Cover and simmer 2 minutes or until tomatoes are soft. Season with salt and pepper. Garnish with parsley. *Makes 6 servings*

Desserts
Contents

Living Without Gluten

Eliminating gluten from your life is not easy, nor is it a short-term proposition. There is no pill for gluten intolerance and no treatment other than changing your diet for good. On the other hand, feeling healthy and energetic for the first time in years can be a huge reward for the effort. At first glance, the list of what you must give up can seem daunting—pasta, bread, crackers, bagels, pretzels, pizza, donuts, even chicken nuggets! The good news is that there are many more foods on the gluten-free list than on the forbidden one. There are also more products, from cereals to baking mixes to pastas, which are now being formulated in gluten-free versions.

Eating gluten-free can mean eating a healthier diet—more fruits and vegetables, less processed food. You may be forced out of your old routine into doing more cooking at home and trying out new ingredients. With a bit of help from the recipes in this book, you just might find your new life is full of delicious surprises.

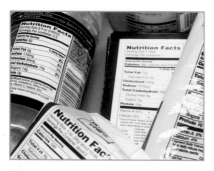

Becoming a Label Detective

Going gluten-free means you will learn a great deal about the many ingredients that go into all the processed food most of us take for granted. You may even decide that paying attention to the ingredients list is a lot more relevant than some of the marketing hype that appears on the front of the package.

The red flag you're searching for is the word "wheat." If anything in the product contains, or is made from wheat, by law it must be listed as such. Next, look for any ingredients you don't recognize. Chances are you'll find a few multisyllabic words that sound like they came from the chemistry lab. You'll need to check a list of safe and unsafe ingredients to figure those out. (You can even download such lists for your smart phone these days. See www.celiac.com for information.) You'll soon recognize the most common ones that can be a problem, even if you never do learn how to pronounce them!

Supermarket Savvy

Before you rush off to buy a cupboard full of specialty products, remember that most basic ingredients are naturally gluten-free. You can pick up fresh produce, meat or fish without worrying. However, frozen dinners and fish sticks are no longer on your list. This doesn't mean you can't have your favorite foods anymore. It just means you will be making some adjustments.

Impulse shopping isn't a great option either. Most supermarkets stock huge displays with brightly colored boxes of highly processed, gluten-filled items. It may also amaze you how many aisles you can skip when you no longer wander aimlessly amidst the latest bread, cracker and snack items.

Of course, you will want to stock up on certain things so that you're prepared to eat well on your new diet. Five years ago a health food store was the only place to buy specialty flours and mixes. Fortunately, today most supermarkets offer just about everything you need.

The Gluten-Free Pantry

Cooking gluten-free is easier if you keep these staples on hand.

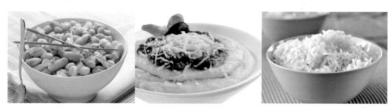

- ❏ beans and lentils
- ❏ chickpea flour
- ❏ corn grits
- ❏ cornmeal and cornstarch
- ❏ corn tortillas and taco shells
- ❏ GF cereal (corn and/or rice)
- ❏ GF flour blends (page 206)
- ❏ GF mixes for your favorite brownies, cookies or muffins
- ❏ GF pasta in various shapes

- ❏ GF soy sauce
- ❏ polenta
- ❏ quinoa
- ❏ rice (arborio rice, basmati rice)
- ❏ rice flour (brown, white and sweet rice flour
- ❏ rice noodles
- ❏ tapioca flour
- ❏ wild rice
- ❏ xanthan gum

Sweet Treats

Orange Granita

. . . .

6 small Valencia or blood oranges
¼ cup sugar
¼ cup water
⅛ teaspoon ground cinnamon

1. Cut oranges in half; squeeze juice into medium bowl and reserve empty shells. Strain juice to remove seeds if necessary. Combine sugar and water in small microwavable bowl; microwave on HIGH 30 seconds to 1 minute or until sugar is dissolved. Stir sugar mixture and cinnamon into juice.

2. Pour juice mixture into shallow 9-inch pan. Cover and place on flat surface in freezer. After 1 to 2 hours when ice crystals form at edges, stir with fork. Stir 2 or 3 more times at 20 to 30 minute intervals until texture of granita is like icy snow.

3. Scoop granita into orange shells to serve.   *Makes 6 servings*

Variation: Add a small amount of orange liqueur to the orange juice mixture before freezing.

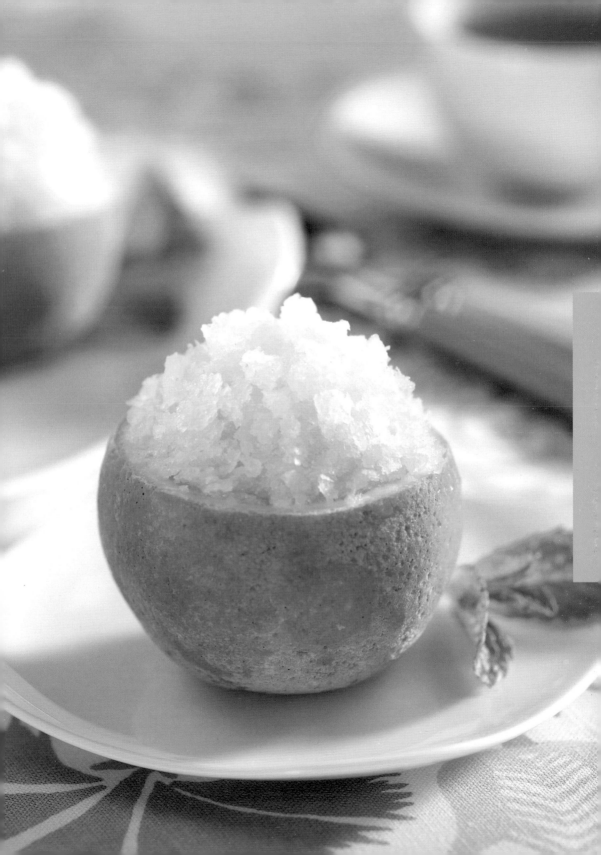

Summer Fruit Brunch Cake

¾ **cup Gluten-Free All-Purpose Flour Blend (recipe follows)***
½ **cup cornmeal**
 1 **teaspoon xanthan gum**
½ **teaspoon baking powder**
¼ **teaspoon baking soda**
⅔ **cup sugar**
½ **cup (1 stick) dairy-free margarine, softened**
 2 **eggs**
½ **cup vanilla soy yogurt, plus additional for topping**
 1 **cup fresh peach slices** *or* **1 can (about 15 ounces) sliced peaches**
    in juice, drained
 Sliced strawberries

*Or use any all-purpose gluten-free flour blend that does not contain xanthan gum.

1. Preheat oven to 325°F. Spray 9-inch pie plate with nonstick cooking spray. Combine flour blend, cornmeal, xanthan gum, baking powder and baking soda in medium bowl.

2. Beat sugar and margarine in large bowl with electric mixer at medium speed until fluffy. Add eggs and ½ cup yogurt; beat until well combined. Beat in flour mixture until combined. Stir in peaches.

3. Pour batter into prepared pie plate. Bake 35 minutes or until toothpick inserted into center comes out clean. Serve with strawberries and drizzle with additional yogurt. *Makes 6 servings*

Gluten-Free All-Purpose Flour Blend: Combine 1 cup white rice flour, 1 cup sorghum flour, 1 cup tapioca flour, 1 cup cornstarch and 1 cup almond or coconut flour in large bowl. Whisk to make sure flours are evenly distributed. The recipe can be doubled or tripled. Store in airtight container in the refrigerator. Makes about 5 cups.

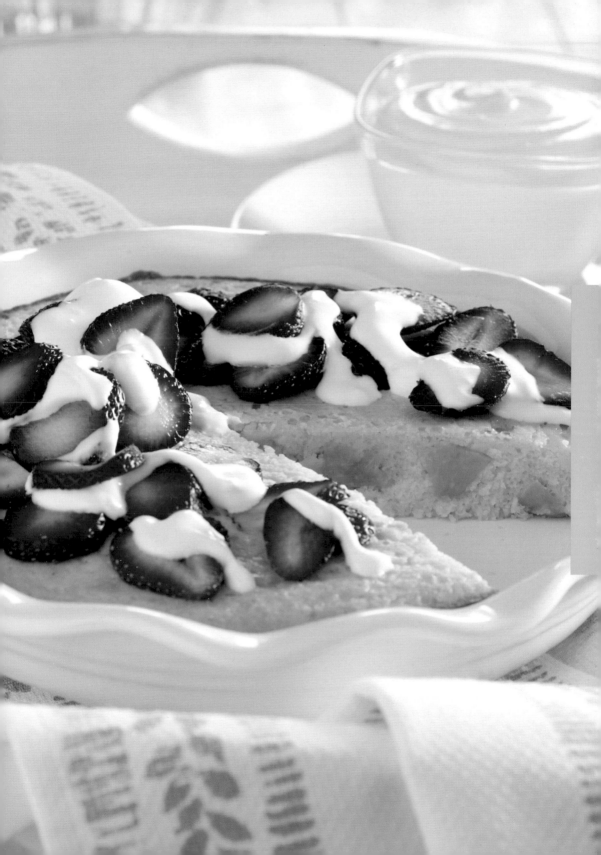

Gluten-Free Apple Pie

Gluten-Free Pie Crust (recipe follows)
6 medium apples, such as Gala, Jonathon or Granny Smith, peeled
  and cut into ¼-inch slices
¾ cup sugar
½ cup dried cranberries
2 tablespoons cornstarch or tapioca flour
2 teaspoons lemon juice
1 teaspoon ground cinnamon

1. Prepare Gluten-Free Pie Crust. Generously butter 9-inch pie pan. Preheat oven to 425°F.

2. Combine apples, sugar, cranberries, cornstarch, lemon juice and cinnamon in large bowl. Toss gently.

3. Press one crust into prepared pan. Arrange apple mixture in crust. Place remaining crust over filling. Pinch edges of crust together; trim excess pastry. Cut slits in top of crust to vent steam.

4. Bake 12 minutes. *Reduce heat to 350°F.* Bake 30 to 40 minutes or until apples feel tender when pierced with tip of sharp knife. Cool on wire rack.

Makes 6 to 8 servings

Gluten-Free Pie Crust

2 cups Gluten-Free All-Purpose Flour Blend (page 108)*
¼ cup sweet rice flour (mochiko)
1 tablespoon sugar
1 teaspoon xanthan gum
½ teaspoon salt
¾ cup (1½ sticks) cold butter
2 eggs
1½ tablespoons cider vinegar

Or use any all-purpose gluten-free flour blend that does not contain xanthan gum.

continued on page 112

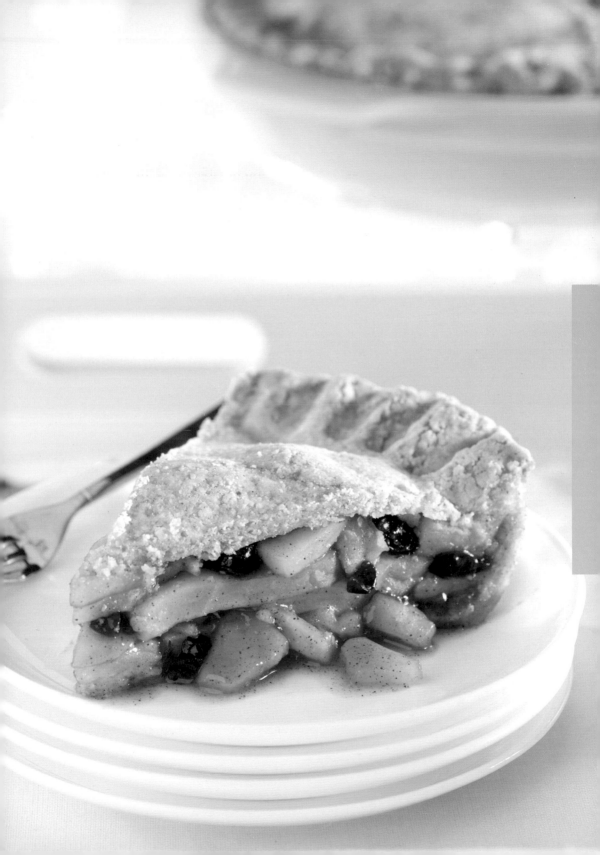

Gluten-Free Pie Crust, continued

1. Mix flour blend, sweet rice flour, sugar, xanthan gum and salt in medium bowl. Cut in butter with pastry blender or two knives until mixture forms coarse crumbs.

2. Make a well in center of mixture. Add eggs and vinegar. Stir together just until dough forms. Divide dough in half; shape into two flat discs. Refrigerate at least 45 minutes or until very cold.

3. Roll each piece of dough on floured surface to circle slightly larger than pie pan. (If dough becomes sticky, return to refrigerator until cold.) Wrap in plastic wrap and refrigerate until ready to use.   *Makes 2 (9-inch) crusts*

Citrus Tapioca Pudding

   2 **navel oranges**
2½ **cups milk**
   ⅓ **cup sugar**
   3 **tablespoons quick-cooking tapioca**
   1 **egg**
   ½ **teaspoon almond extract**
      Ground cinnamon or nutmeg
      Additional orange slices (optional)

1. Grate peel of 1 orange into medium saucepan. Add milk, sugar, tapioca and egg; let stand 5 minutes. Cook and stir over medium heat until mixture comes to a boil. Remove from heat; stir in almond extract. Let stand 20 minutes. Stir well; let cool to room temperature. Cover and refrigerate at least 2 hours.

2. Peel and dice oranges. Stir tapioca mixture; fold in oranges. Spoon into dessert dishes. Sprinkle with cinnamon; garnish with additional orange slices.
                                              Makes 6 servings

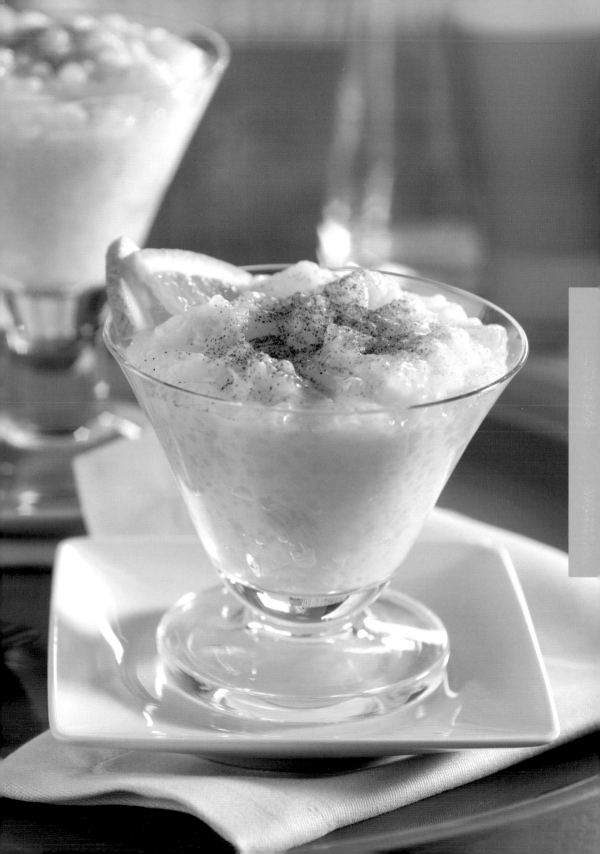

Easy Orange Cake

1½ cups Gluten-Free All-Purpose Flour Blend (page 108)*
½ cup sugar
1 teaspoon baking soda
1 teaspoon xanthan gum
¼ teaspoon salt
   Grated peel of 1 orange
⅔ cup orange juice
5 tablespoons vegetable oil
   Orange No-Butter Buttercream Frosting (recipe follows)

Or use any all-purpose gluten-free flour blend that does not contain xanthan gum.

1. Preheat oven to 350°F. Spray 9-inch round cake pan with nonstick cooking spray.

2. Combine flour blend, sugar, baking soda, xanthan gum, salt and orange peel in medium bowl. Combine orange juice and oil in small bowl or measuring cup. Add wet ingredients to flour mixture and stir until smooth. Spread in prepared pan.

3. Bake 30 minutes or until toothpick inserted into center comes out clean. Meanwhile, prepare Orange No-Butter Buttercream Frosting.

4. Cool cake in pan on wire rack 5 minutes. Remove from pan and cool completely. Frost cake. *Makes 6 servings*

Orange No-Butter Buttercream Frosting

½ cup (1 stick) dairy-free margarine (not spread)
2 teaspoons grated orange peel
2 tablespoons orange juice
1 teaspoon vanilla
4 cups powdered sugar
4 to 6 tablespoons soy creamer

continued on page 116

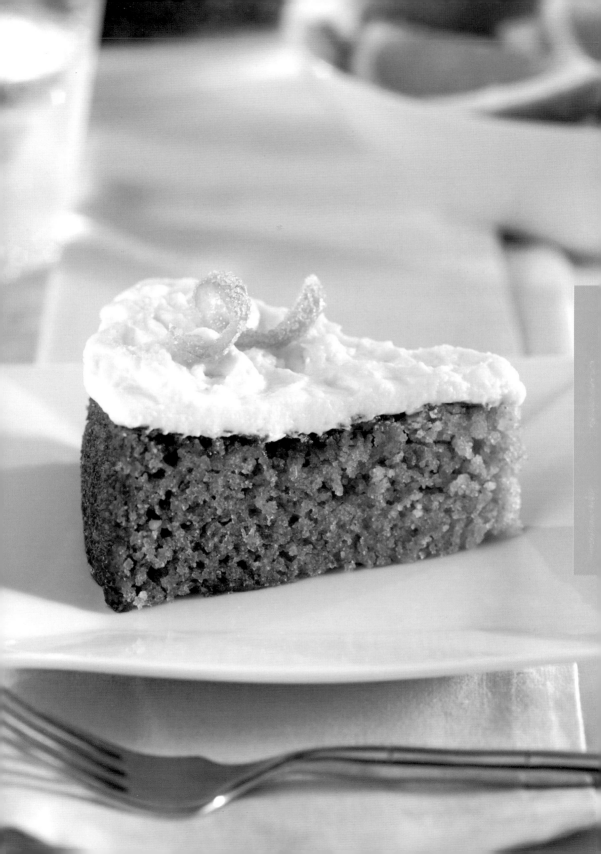

Orange No-Butter Buttercream Frosting, continued

1. Beat margarine in medium bowl with electric mixer at medium speed until light and fluffy. Beat in orange peel, orange juice and vanilla.

2. Gradually beat in powdered sugar. Beat in soy creamer by tablespoonfuls until spreadable.

Mixed Berry Crisp

    6 cups mixed berries, thawed if frozen
    ¾ cup packed brown sugar, divided
    ¼ cup tapioca flour
       Juice of ½ lemon
     1 teaspoon ground cinnamon
    ½ cup rice flour
     6 tablespoons cold butter, cut into small pieces
    ½ cup sliced almonds

1. Preheat oven to 375°F. Grease 8- or 9-inch square baking pan. Combine berries, ¼ cup brown sugar, tapioca flour, lemon juice and cinnamon in large bowl. Transfer to prepared pan.

2. Place rice flour, remaining ½ cup brown sugar and butter in food processor. Process using on/off pulsing action until mixture resembles coarse crumbs. Add almonds; process using on/off pulsing action until combined.

3. Sprinkle almond mixture over berry mixture. Bake 20 to 30 minutes or until golden brown. *Makes 9 servings*

Tip

For a gluten-free fruit dessert, a crisp is considerably easier than a pie since you don't need to bother with making a special crust. This recipe uses tapioca flour as a thickening agent, but you could also use cornstarch or arrowroot.

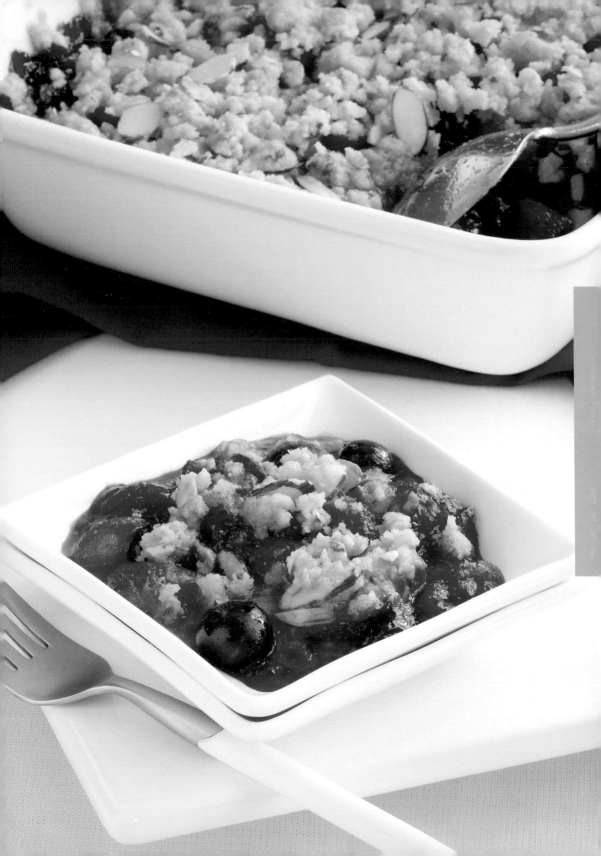

Almond Flour Pound Cake

½ cup (1 stick) butter, softened

4 ounces cream cheese, softened

¾ cup sugar

4 eggs

1 teaspoon vanilla

2 cups almond flour*

1 teaspoon baking powder

½ teaspoon salt

¼ teaspoon ground ginger

¼ teaspoon ground cardamom

1 tablespoon honey roasted sliced almonds

*Almond flour, also called almond meal, is available in the specialty flour section of the supermarket or can be ordered on the Internet.

1. Preheat oven to 350°F. Spray 9×5-inch loaf pan with nonstick cooking spray.

2. Beat butter, cream cheese and sugar in large bowl with electric mixer at medium speed until well blended.

3. Add eggs, one at a time, beating after each addition. Beat in vanilla.

4. Combine almond flour, baking powder, salt, ginger and cardamom in medium bowl. Gradually add to egg mixture, beating until blended.

5. Pour into prepared pan; sprinkle with sliced almonds. Bake 45 to 55 minutes or until toothpick inserted into center comes out clean.   *Makes 9 servings*

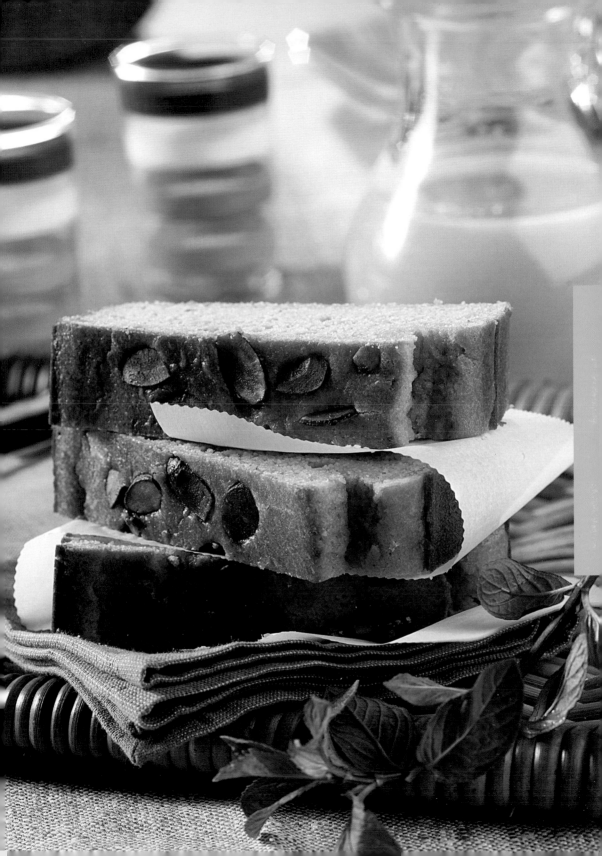

Grilled Peaches with Nutmeg Pastry Cream

4 peaches, halved
Cinnamon-sugar*
3 egg yolks
⅓ cup sugar
2 tablespoons sweet rice flour (mochiko)
Pinch salt
1¼ cups whole milk
1 teaspoon vanilla
⅛ teaspoon ground nutmeg
2 tablespoons butter
Whipped cream (optional)

To make cinnamon-sugar, combine 2 tablespoons sugar with 1 teaspoon ground cinnamon.

1. Prepare grill for direct cooking. Sprinkle peach halves with cinnamon-sugar. Grill over medium-low heat just until tender. (Peaches should still be firm and hold shape.) Set aside.

2. Combine egg yolks, sugar, sweet rice flour and salt in medium bowl until well blended.

3. Bring milk, vanilla and nutmeg to a boil in medium saucepan over medium-low heat. Whisking constantly, slowly add ¼ cup hot milk mixture to egg yolk mixture.

4. Add egg yolk mixture to milk mixture in saucepan; cook, whisking constantly, until thickened. Remove from heat and add butter; whisk until well blended.

5. Spoon sauce onto dessert plates; arrange peach halves on top of sauce. Serve with whipped cream, if desired.   *Makes 4 servings*

Sweet Treats

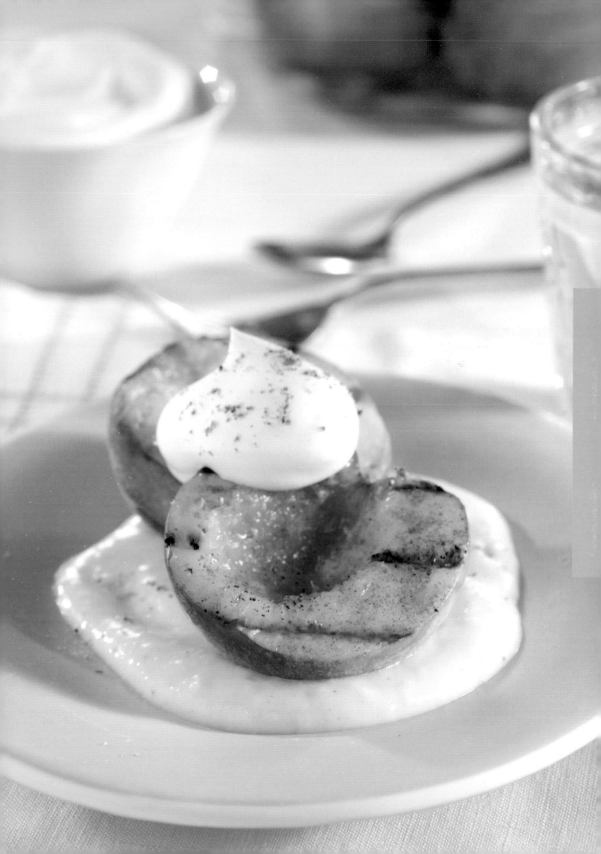

Carrot-Spice Snack Cake

½ **cup packed brown sugar**
⅓ **cup dairy-free margarine**
2 **eggs**
½ **cup soymilk or other milk**
1 **teaspoon vanilla**
1¼ **cups Gluten-Free All-Purpose Flour Blend (page 108)***
¾ **cup finely shredded carrot**
2 **teaspoons baking powder**
1½ **teaspoons pumpkin pie spice**
½ **teaspoon xanthan gum**
½ **teaspoon salt**
⅓ **cup golden raisins**
Powdered sugar

*Or use any all-purpose gluten-free flour blend that does not contain xanthan gum.

1. Preheat oven to 350°F. Spray 8-inch square baking pan with nonstick cooking spray.

2. Beat brown sugar and margarine in medium bowl with electric mixer at medium speed until well blended. Beat in eggs, soymilk and vanilla.

3. Stir in flour blend, carrot, baking powder, pumpkin pie spice, xanthan gum and salt. Stir in raisins.

4. Spread batter in prepared pan. Bake 25 to 30 minutes or until toothpick inserted into center comes out clean. Cool completely in pan on wire rack. Just before serving, sprinkle with powdered sugar.   *Makes 8 servings*

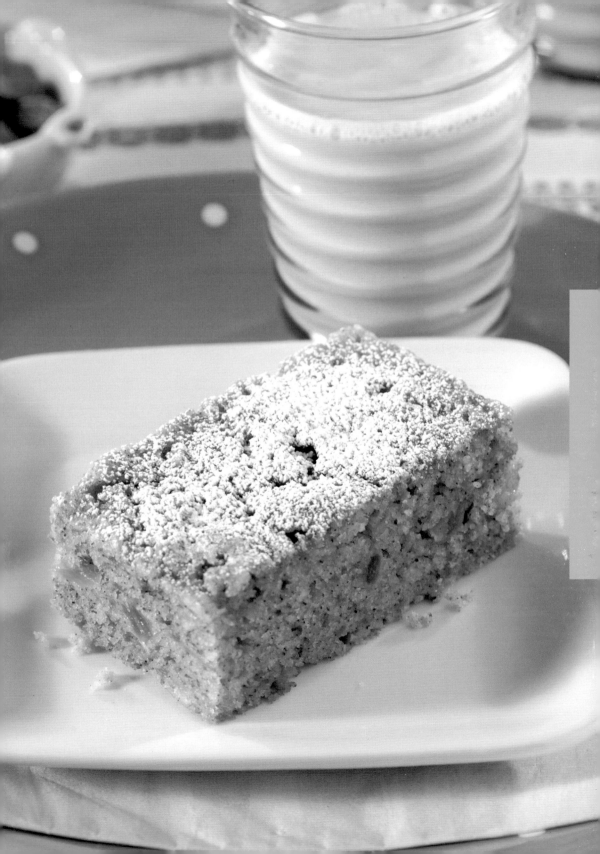

Mochi Rice Cake Rainbow

1 cup sweet rice flour (mochiko)*
¾ cup sugar
⅔ cup tapioca flour
Pinch salt
1 can (13½ ounces) unsweetened coconut milk
¼ to ½ cup water
Assorted paste food coloring

*Sweet rice flour is usually labeled mochiko (the Japanese term). It is available in the Asian section of large supermarkets, at Asian grocers and on the Internet.

1. Spray 8×4-inch loaf pan or four 8-ounce custard cups with nonstick cooking spray. Set up steamer large enough to hold pan or cups over large saucepan of water.

2. Combine sweet rice flour, sugar, tapioca flour and salt in large bowl. Add coconut milk and whisk to combine. Whisk in water by tablespoons until batter is smooth with consistency of heavy cream.

3. Divide batter into 3 or 4 medium bowls or measuring cups. Add different food coloring to each bowl and whisk to blend completely. Bring water in saucepan to a boil.

4. Pour one layer of colored batter into prepared pan. (This color will be on top of finished mochi.) Place pan in steamer; cover and reduce heat to a simmer. Steam about 8 minutes or until mochi is set in center. Carefully uncover steamer and gently touch center of mochi to check doneness.

5. Pour second color of batter over first color. Layers can be as thick or thin as desired. Cover and steam 8 minutes or until second layer is set. Proceed with remaining batter, steaming each layer until set. Make as many layers as desired until all of batter is used.

6. When final layer is set, remove pan from steamer and cool. Refrigerate at least 1 hour or until ready to serve. Loosen sides of mochi from pan and invert onto serving dish. It is easiest to slice mochi with a plastic knife.

Makes 6 to 8 servings

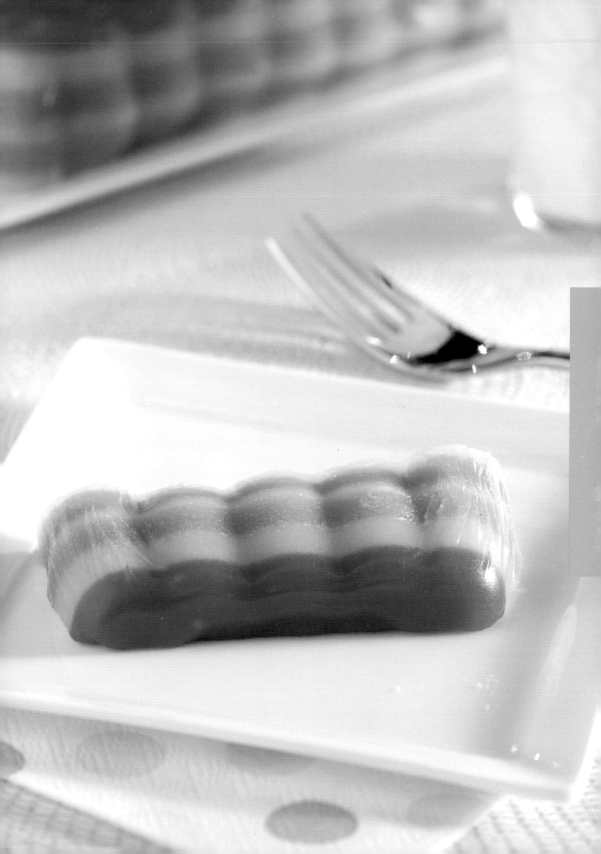

Chocolate Rules

Cocoa Bottom Banana Pecan Bars

1 cup sugar
½ cup (1 stick) dairy-free margarine
5 ripe bananas, mashed
1 egg
1 teaspoon vanilla
1½ cups Gluten-Free All-Purpose Flour Blend (page 108)*
1 teaspoon baking powder
1 teaspoon baking soda
½ teaspoon xanthan gum
½ teaspoon salt
½ cup chopped pecans
¼ cup unsweetened cocoa powder

Or use any all-purpose gluten-free flour blend that does not contain xanthan gum.

1. Preheat oven to 350°F. Grease 13×9-inch baking pan.

2. Beat sugar and margarine in large bowl with electric mixer at medium speed until creamy. Add bananas, egg and vanilla; beat until well blended. Combine flour blend, baking powder, baking soda, xanthan gum and salt in medium bowl. Add to banana mixture; beat until well blended. Stir in pecans.

3. Remove half of batter to another bowl; stir in cocoa. Spread chocolate batter in prepared pan. Top with plain batter; swirl with knife.

4. Bake 30 to 35 minutes or until edges are lightly browned. Cool completely in pan on wire rack. Cut into bars.   *Makes 2 dozen bars*

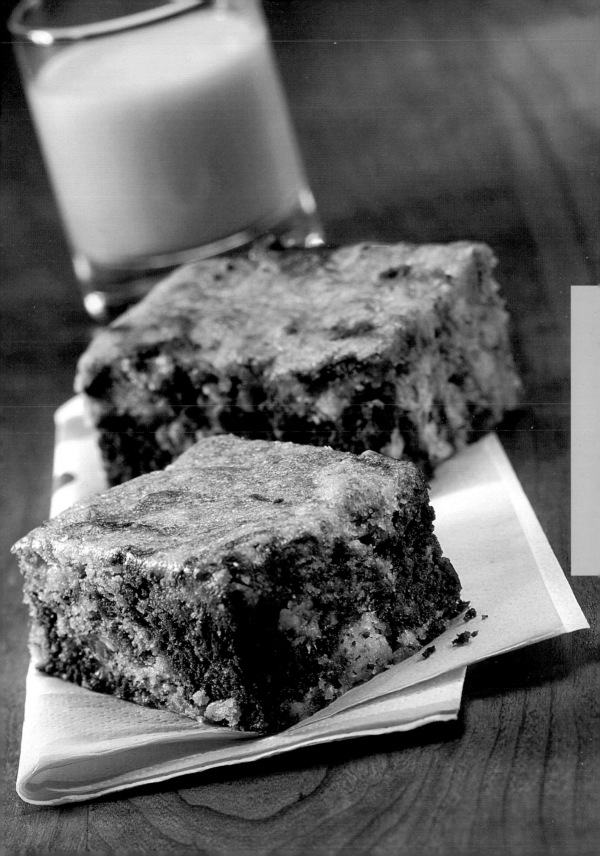

Chocolate Macarons

1 cup powdered sugar

⅔ cup blanched almond flour*

3 tablespoons unsweetened cocoa powder

3 egg whites, at room temperature**

¼ cup granulated sugar

Chocolate-hazelnut spread or raspberry jam

Blanched almond flour, also called almond powder, is available in the specialty flour section of the supermarket or can be ordered on the Internet.

**For best results, separate the eggs while cold. Leave the egg whites at room temperature for 3 or 4 hours. Reserve yolks in refrigerator for another use.*

1. Line two baking sheets with parchment paper. Double baking sheets by placing another sheet underneath each to protect macarons from burning or cracking. (Do NOT use insulated baking sheets.)

2. Place powdered sugar, almond flour and cocoa in food processor. Pulse 2 to 3 minutes or until well combined into very fine powder, scraping bowl occasionally. Sift mixture twice. Discard any remaining large pieces.

3. Beat egg whites in large bowl with electric mixer at high speed until foamy. Gradually add granulated sugar, beating at high speed 2 to 3 minutes or until mixture forms stiff, shiny peaks, scraping bowl occasionally.

4. Add half of sifted flour mixture to egg whites. Stir with spatula to combine (about 12 strokes). Repeat with remaining flour mixture. Mix about 15 strokes more by pressing against side of bowl and scooping from bottom until batter is smooth and shiny. Check consistency by dropping spoonful of batter onto plate. It should have a peak which quickly relaxes back into batter. *Do not overmix or undermix.*

5. Attach ½-inch plain piping tip to pastry bag. Scoop batter into bag. Pipe 1-inch circles onto prepared baking sheet about 2 inches apart. Rap baking sheet on flat surface to remove air bubbles and set aside. Repeat with remaining batter. Let macarons rest, uncovered, until tops harden slightly; this takes from 15 minutes on dry days to 1 hour in more humid conditions. Gently touch top of macaron to check. When batter does not stick, macarons are ready to bake.

continued on page 130

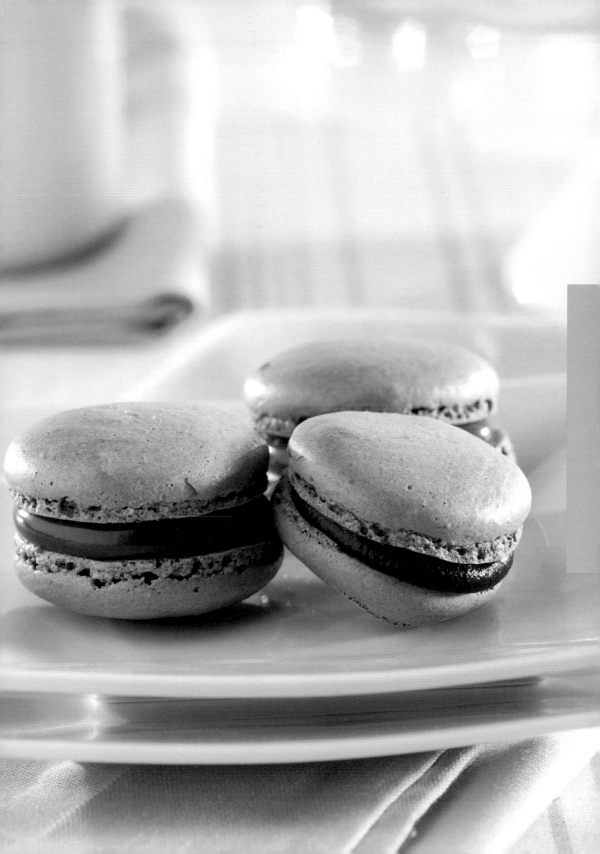

6. Meanwhile, preheat oven to 375°F. Place oven rack in center. Place 1 baking sheet of macarons in oven. *After 5 minutes reduce heat to 325°F.* Bake 10 to 13 minutes, checking at 5 minute intervals. If macarons begin to brown, cover loosely with foil and reduce oven temperature or prop oven open slightly with wooden spoon. Repeat with remaining baking sheet.

7. Cool completely on pan on wire rack. While cooling, if they appear to be sticking to parchment, lift parchment edges and spray pan underneath lightly with water. Steam will help release macarons.

8. Match same size cookies and fill with chocolate-hazelnut spread. Store macarons in covered container in refrigerator for 4 or 5 days. Freeze for longer storage. *Makes 16 to 20 macaron sandwiches*

Microwave Chocolate Pudding

¼ cup unsweetened cocoa powder
2 tablespoons cornstarch
1½ cups milk
⅓ cup sugar
1 teaspoon vanilla
⅛ teaspoon ground cinnamon

1. Combine cocoa and cornstarch in medium microwavable bowl or 1-quart glass measure. Gradually whisk in milk until well blended.

2. Microwave on HIGH 2 minutes; stir. Microwave on MEDIUM-HIGH (70%) 3½ to 4½ minutes or until thickened, stirring every 1½ minutes.

3. Stir in sugar, vanilla and cinnamon. Let stand at least 5 minutes before serving, stirring occasionally to prevent skin from forming. Serve warm or chilled. *Makes 4 servings*

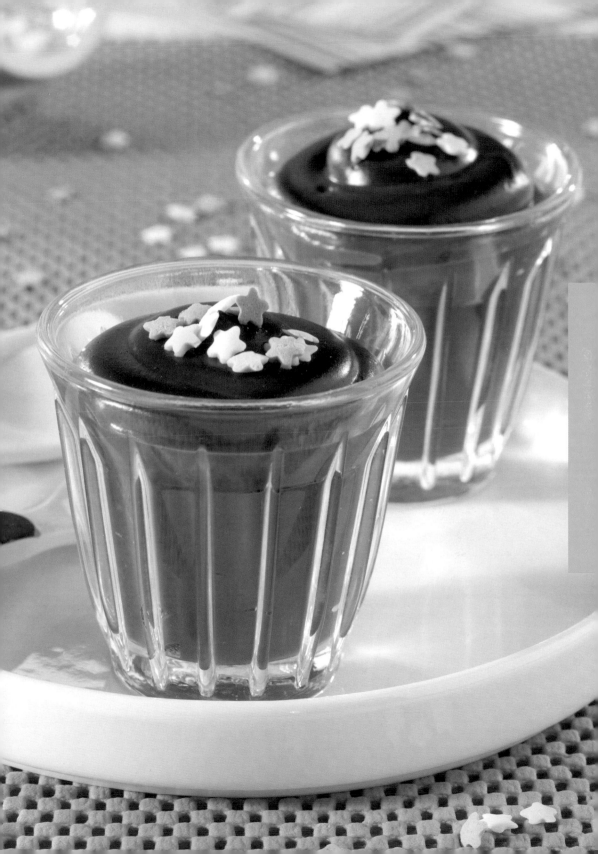

Flourless Chocolate Cake

3 squares (1 ounce each) semisweet chocolate, chopped
3 tablespoons butter
1 tablespoon espresso powder or instant coffee granules
2 tablespoons hot water
4 eggs, separated
2 egg whites
⅔ cup sugar, divided
3 tablespoons unsweetened cocoa powder, sifted
1 teaspoon vanilla
½ teaspoon salt
Whipped cream and raspberries (optional)

1. Preheat oven to 300°F. Grease 9-inch springform pan; line bottom of pan with parchment paper.

2. Melt chocolate and butter in small heavy saucepan over low heat, stirring frequently; cool. Dissolve espresso powder in hot water in small bowl.

3. Place 6 egg whites in large bowl; set aside. Beat egg yolks in medium bowl with electric mixer at high speed about 5 minutes or until pale yellow in color. Add ⅓ cup sugar; beat about 4 minutes or until mixture falls in ribbons from beaters. Slowly beat in melted chocolate mixture and espresso mixture at low speed. Beat in cocoa and vanilla just until blended.

4. Add salt to egg whites; beat at high speed 2 minutes or until soft peaks form. Beat in remaining ⅓ cup sugar until stiff peaks form. Stir large spoonful of egg whites into chocolate mixture. Fold chocolate mixture into egg whites until almost blended. Spoon batter into prepared pan.

5. Bake 1 hour or until cake begins to pull away from side of pan. Cool on wire rack 10 minutes; run thin spatula around edge of cake. Carefully remove side of pan. Cool completely. Invert cake; remove bottom of pan and paper from cake. Cover and refrigerate at least 4 hours. Serve chilled with whipped cream and raspberries, if desired. *Makes 10 servings*

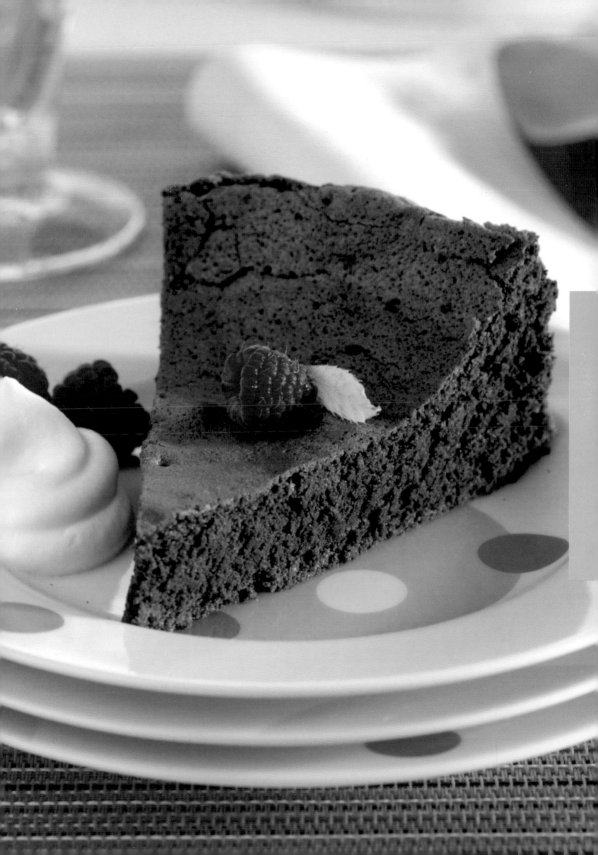

Gluten-Free Fudge Cookies

2 packages (12 ounces each) semisweet chocolate chips, divided
½ cup (1 stick) butter, cut into chunks
2 eggs
1 teaspoon vanilla
¾ cup plus 2 tablespoons sugar
⅔ cup Gluten-Free All-Purpose Flour Blend (page 108)*
2 tablespoons unsweetened Dutch process cocoa powder
1 teaspoon baking powder
½ teaspoon xanthan gum
¼ teaspoon salt

*Or use any all-purpose gluten-free flour blend that does not contain xanthan gum.

1. Line cookie sheets with parchment paper.

2. Combine 1 package chocolate chips and butter in large microwavable bowl. Microwave on HIGH 30 seconds; stir. Repeat as necessary until chips are melted and mixture is smooth. Let cool slightly.

3. Beat eggs and vanilla in large bowl with electric mixer at medium speed until blended and frothy. Add sugar; beat until thick. Add chocolate mixture; beat until well blended. Add flour blend, cocoa, baking powder, xanthan gum and salt; beat until combined. Stir in remaining chocolate chips.

4. Drop dough by rounded tablespoonfuls 1½ inches apart onto prepared cookie sheets. Refrigerate 30 minutes.

5. Preheat oven to 325°F. Bake 16 to 20 minutes or until cookies are firm. Cool on cookie sheets 2 minutes. Remove to wire racks; cool completely.

Makes about 2½ dozen cookies

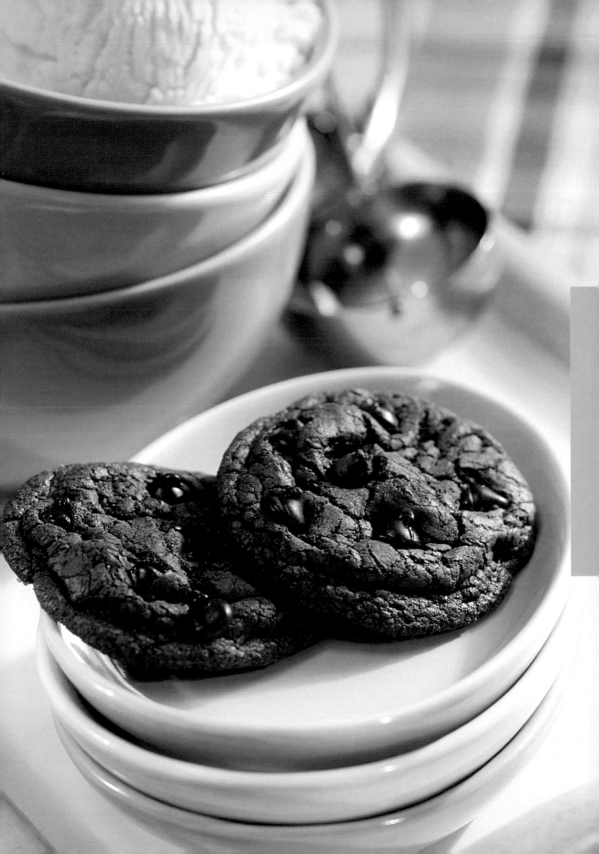

Mini Swirl Cheesecakes

8 squares (1 ounce each) semisweet baking chocolate
3 packages (8 ounces each) cream cheese, softened
½ cup sugar
3 eggs
1 teaspoon vanilla

1. Preheat oven to 325°F. Lightly grease 12 standard (2½-inch) muffin cups.

2. Place chocolate in 1-cup microwavable bowl. Microwave on HIGH 1 to 1½ minutes or until chocolate is melted, stirring after 1 minute. Let cool slightly.

3. Beat cream cheese and sugar in large bowl with electric mixer at medium speed about 2 minutes or until light and fluffy. Add eggs and vanilla; beat about 2 minutes or until well blended. Place about 2 heaping tablespoons of mixture in each muffin cup.

4. Beat melted chocolate into remaining cream cheese mixture until well blended. Spoon chocolate mixture on top of plain mixture in muffin cups. Swirl batter with knife.

5. Place muffin pan in larger baking pan; place in oven. Pour warm water into larger pan to depth of ½ to 1 inch. Bake 30 minutes or until edges are dry and centers are almost set. Remove muffin pan from water. Cool cheesecakes completely in muffin pan on wire rack. *Makes 12 mini cheesecakes*

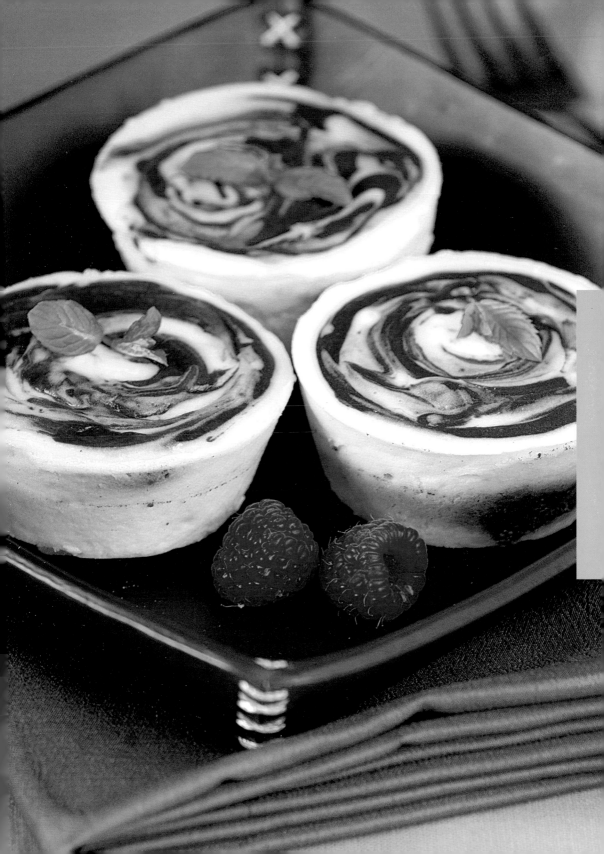

Chocolate Cupcakes

2½ **cups Gluten-Free All-Purpose Flour Blend (page 108)***

½ **cup unsweetened cocoa powder**

1½ **teaspoons baking soda**

¾ **teaspoon xanthan gum**

½ **teaspoon baking powder**

¼ **teaspoon salt**

1½ **cups sugar**

3 **eggs**

½ **cup vegetable oil**

1 **teaspoon vanilla**

1¼ **cups plain soymilk or other milk**

Creamy White Frosting (page 138)

Or use any all-purpose gluten-free flour blend that does not contain xanthan gum.

1. Preheat oven to 350°F. Line 18 standard (2½-inch) muffin cups with paper baking cups.

2. Mix flour blend, cocoa, baking soda, xanthan gum, baking powder and salt in large bowl. Beat sugar, eggs, oil and vanilla in large bowl with electric mixer at medium speed 3 minutes or until thick and smooth.

3. Add flour mixture and soymilk alternately to sugar mixture, beating at low speed and scraping side and bottom of bowl occasionally. Beat at medium speed 2 minutes.

4. Fill prepared muffin cups two-thirds full. Bake 20 to 25 minutes or until toothpick inserted into centers comes out clean. Cool in pans on wire racks 5 minutes. Remove from pans; cool completely.

5. Meanwhile, prepare Creamy White Frosting. Frost cupcakes.

Makes 18 cupcakes

continued on page 140

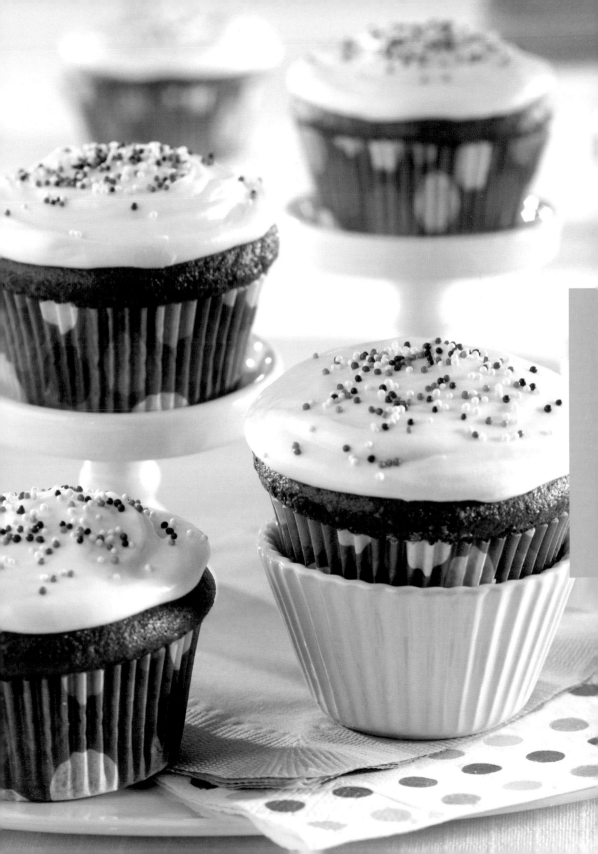

Creamy White Frosting

....

4 ounces dairy-free cream cheese alternative
3 tablespoons dairy-free margarine
1½ teaspoons vanilla
4 to 5 cups powdered sugar
4 to 6 tablespoons soymilk or other milk

Beat cream cheese alternative and margarine in medium bowl with electric mixer at medium speed until light and fluffy. Beat in vanilla. Gradually beat in powdered sugar. Beat in soymilk by tablespoonfuls until spreadable.

Cocoa Chewies

....

⅓ cup powdered sugar
2 tablespoons flaked coconut
2 tablespoons unsweetened cocoa powder
1 tablespoon cornstarch
3 egg whites
½ teaspoon vanilla
¼ cup granulated sugar

1. Preheat oven to 250°F. Line baking sheets with parchment paper or foil.

2. Combine powdered sugar, coconut, cocoa and cornstarch in small bowl. Beat egg whites and vanilla in medium bowl with electric mixer at high speed until foamy. Gradually add granulated sugar, 1 tablespoon at a time, beating until stiff peaks form. Gently fold in coconut mixture. Pipe or spoon egg white mixture into scant 2-inch mounds onto prepared baking sheets.

3. Bake 1 hour. Cool cookies completely on baking sheets.

Makes 2 dozen cookies

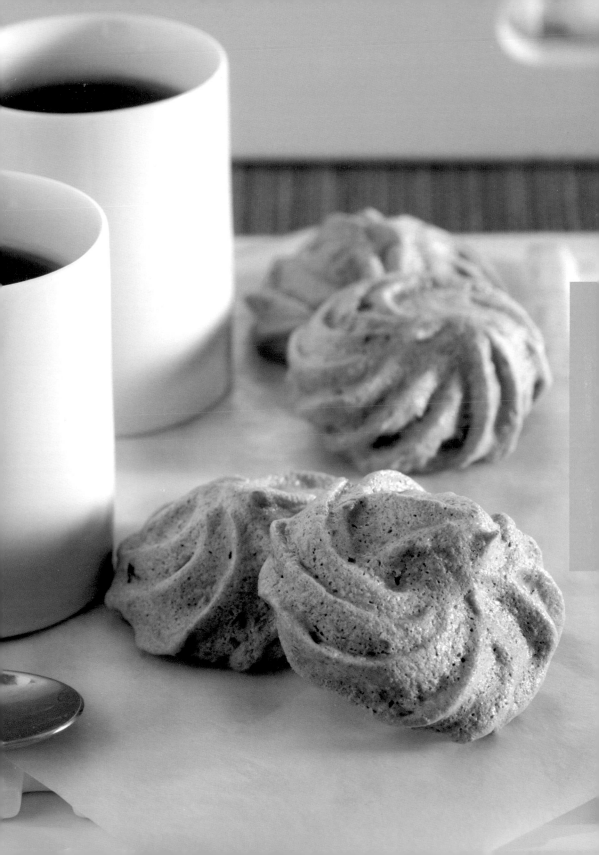

Chocolate Crème Brulée

2 cups whipping cream
3 squares (1 ounce each) semisweet baking chocolate, finely chopped
3 egg yolks
¼ cup granulated sugar
2 teaspoons vanilla
3 tablespoons packed brown sugar

1. Preheat oven to 325°F. Heat cream in medium saucepan over medium heat until it just begins to simmer. *Do not boil.* Remove from heat; stir in chocolate until melted and smooth. Set aside to cool slightly.

2. Beat egg yolks and granulated sugar in large bowl with electric mixer at medium-high speed 5 minutes or until thick and pale yellow. Beat in chocolate mixture and vanilla until blended.

3. Divide mixture among four 6-ounce custard cups or individual baking dishes. Place cups in baking pan; place pan in oven. Pour boiling water into baking pan to reach halfway up sides of custard cups. Cover loosely with foil.

4. Bake 30 minutes or until edges are just set. Remove cups from baking pan to wire rack to cool completely. Wrap with plastic wrap and refrigerate 4 hours or up to 3 days.

5. When ready to serve, preheat broiler. Spread about 2 teaspoons brown sugar evenly over each cup. Broil 3 to 4 minutes or until sugar bubbles and browns, watching carefully. Serve immediately. *Makes 4 servings*

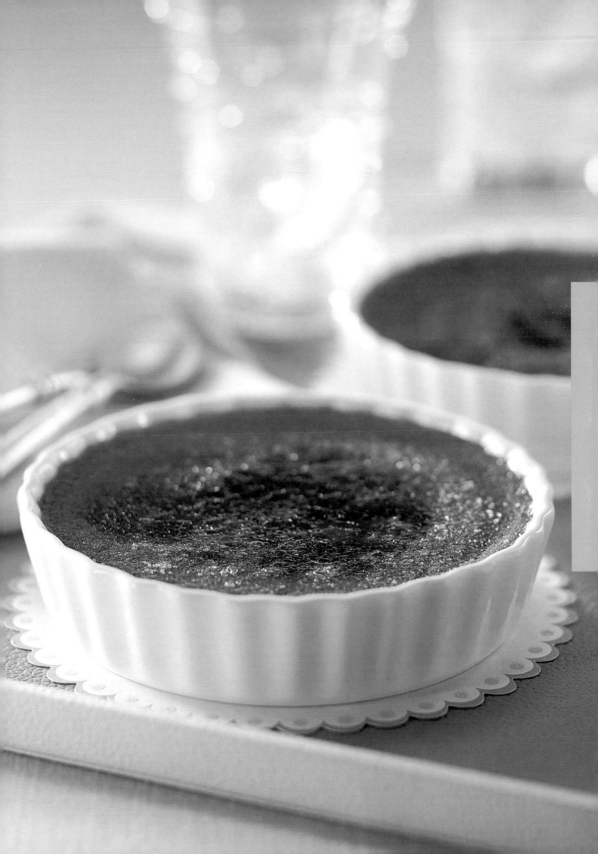

No-Wheat Brownies

¼ **cup cornstarch**

¼ **cup brown rice flour**

1 **teaspoon baking soda**

¼ **teaspoon salt**

½ **cup (1 stick) dairy-free margarine**

1 **cup packed brown sugar**

½ **cup unsweetened cocoa powder**

½ **cup semisweet chocolate chips**

1 **teaspoon vanilla**

2 **eggs, lightly beaten**

    Sliced strawberries (optional)

1. Preheat oven to 350°F. Spray 8-inch square baking pan with nonstick cooking spray. Mix cornstarch, rice flour, baking soda and salt in small bowl.

2. Melt margarine in large saucepan over low heat. Add brown sugar; cook and stir about 4 minutes or until sugar is completely dissolved and mixture is smooth. Remove from heat; sift in cocoa and stir until combined. Add flour mixture and stir until smooth. (Mixture will be thick.)

3. Stir in chocolate chips and vanilla. Beat in eggs until mixture is smooth. Spoon batter into prepared pan.

4. Bake 25 to 30 minutes or until toothpick inserted into center comes out almost clean. Garnish with strawberries.

Makes 9 brownies

Tip

Brownies and fudgy cookies usually bake up well in gluten-free forms. They don't require much flour and they are dense by nature. This brownie recipe doesn't even require any xanthan gum since it doesn't need to rise or puff up. And strong flavors like chocolate help mask any off tastes from gluten-free flours.

Chocolate Rules

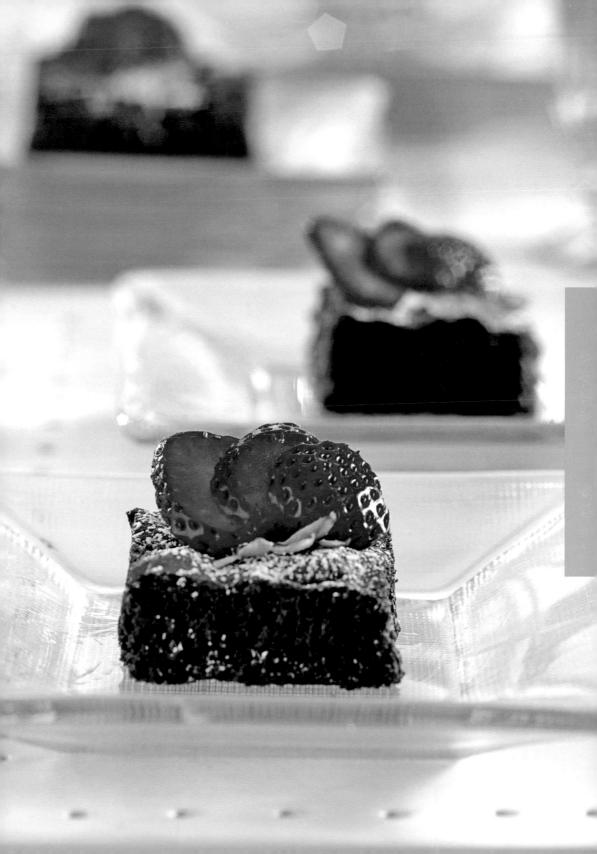

Safe Kid Stuff

Banana & Chocolate Chip Pops

1 small ripe banana
1 container (6 ounces) banana yogurt
⅛ teaspoon ground nutmeg
2 tablespoons mini chocolate chips
4 (3-ounce) paper cups and wooden sticks

1. Slice banana; place in food processor with yogurt and nutmeg. Process until smooth. Transfer to small bowl; stir in chocolate chips.

2. Spoon banana mixture into paper cups. Freeze 1 hour, then insert wooden sticks. Freeze completely. Peel cups off pops to serve.   *Makes 4 servings*

Peanut Butter & Jelly Pops: Stir ¼ cup peanut butter in small bowl until smooth; stir in 1 container (6 ounces) vanilla yogurt. Drop 2 tablespoons strawberry preserves on top of mixture; pull spoon back and forth through mixture several times to swirl slightly. Spoon into cups and freeze as directed above. Makes 4 servings.

Blueberry-Lime Pops: Stir 1 container (6 ounces) Key lime yogurt in small bowl until smooth; fold in ⅓ cup frozen blueberries. Spoon into cups and freeze as directed above. Makes 4 servings.

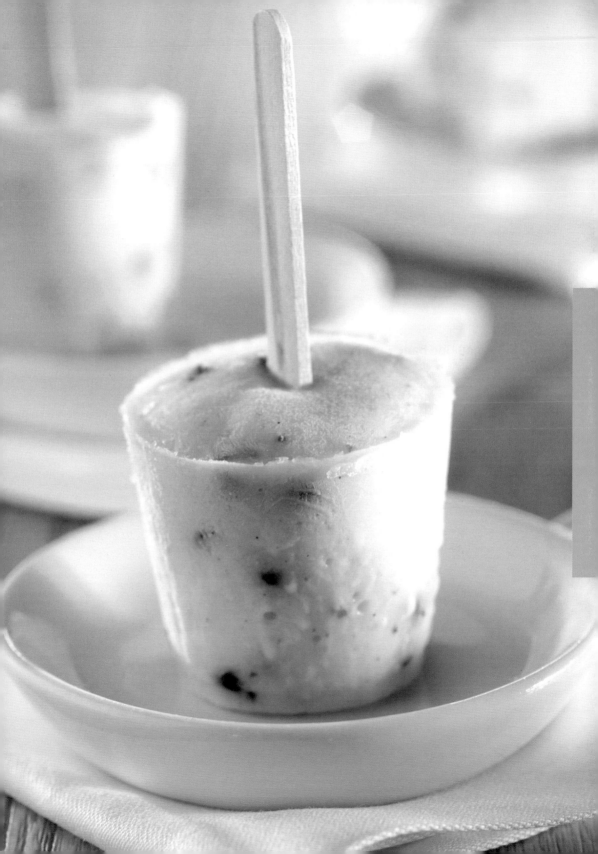

Very Orange Cake

....

1 package (15 ounces) gluten-free yellow cake mix
⅔ cup orange juice
½ cup (1 stick) dairy-free margarine
3 eggs
1 teaspoon vanilla
1 package (4-serving size) orange gelatin
½ cup boiling water
¼ cup cold water
Marshmallow Frosting (recipe follows)
Candy orange slices (optional)

1. Preheat oven to 350°F. Spray 8-inch square cake pan with nonstick cooking spray.

2. Combine cake mix, orange juice, margarine, eggs and vanilla in large bowl. Beat with electric mixer at low speed 30 seconds to combine. Beat at medium speed 2 minutes or until smooth. Pour batter into prepared pan.

3. Bake 40 to 50 minutes or until toothpick inserted into center comes out almost clean. Cool in pan on wire rack.

4. Place half of orange gelatin powder in small bowl or measuring cup. (Discard remaining powder.) Stir ½ cup boiling water into gelatin until completely dissolved. Stir in ¼ cup cold water. Poke cake at ½-inch intervals with fork or skewer. Pour gelatin mixture over cake. Refrigerate 2 to 3 hours or until firm.

5. Meanwhile, prepare Marshmallow Frosting. Frost cake and decorate with candy orange slices. *Makes 12 to 16 servings*

Marshmallow Frosting: Combine 1 package (8 ounces) cream cheese, 1 jar (7 ounces) marshmallow creme and 1 teaspoon vanilla in large bowl. Beat with electric mixer at medium speed until fluffy.

Safe Kid Stuff

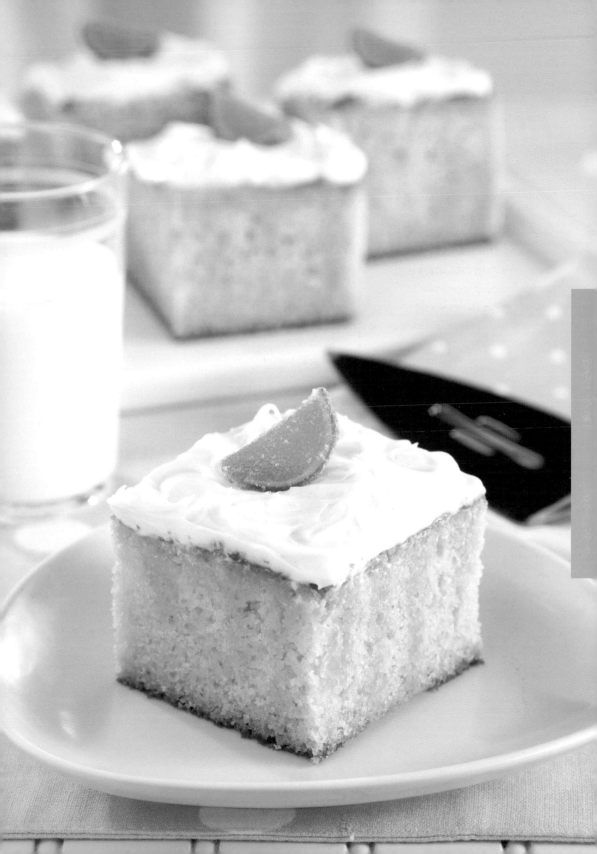

One-Bite Pineapple Chewies

½ **cup whipping cream**
¼ **cup sugar**
⅛ **teaspoon salt**
1 **cup finely chopped dried pineapple**
½ **cup coarsely chopped slivered almonds**
¼ **cup mini semisweet chocolate chips**
¼ **cup white rice flour**

1. Preheat oven to 350°F. Line two cookie sheets with parchment paper.

2. Stir cream, sugar and salt in large bowl until sugar dissolves. Stir in pineapple, almonds and chocolate chips. Stir in rice flour until blended.

3. Drop dough by rounded teaspoonfuls about 1 inch apart onto prepared cookie sheets. Bake 13 to 15 minutes or until edges are golden brown. Cool on cookie sheets 2 minutes. Remove to wire racks to cool completely.

Makes about 1½ dozen cookies

Tip

Rice flour should be a staple in your gluten-free pantry. It is virtually tasteless and reasonably priced. Use it to "flour" foods or baking surfaces in place of wheat flour. In small quantities, as in this recipe, rice flour can stand in for wheat flour.

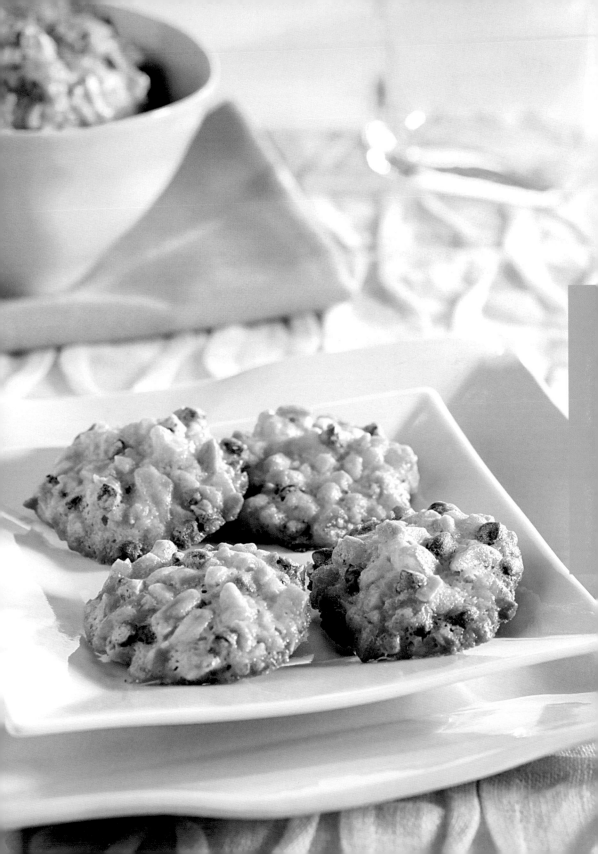

Magic Rainbow Pops

1 envelope (¼ ounce) unflavored gelatin
¼ cup cold water
½ cup boiling water
1 container (6 ounces) raspberry or strawberry yogurt
1 container (6 ounces) lemon or orange yogurt
1 can (8¼ ounces) apricots or peaches with juice
Pop molds

1. Combine gelatin and cold water in 2-cup glass measuring cup. Let stand 5 minutes to soften. Add boiling water. Stir until gelatin is completely dissolved. Cool.

2. For first layer, combine raspberry yogurt and ¼ cup gelatin mixture in small bowl; stir until completely blended. Fill each pop mold about one third full with raspberry mixture.* Freeze 30 to 60 minutes or until set.

3. For second layer, combine lemon yogurt and ¼ cup gelatin mixture in small bowl; stir until completely blended. Pour lemon mixture over raspberry layer in each mold.* Freeze 30 to 60 minutes or until set.

4. For third layer, place apricots with juice and remaining ¼ cup gelatin mixture in blender. Process 20 seconds or until smooth. Pour apricot mixture into each mold.* Cover each pop with mold top; freeze 2 to 5 hours or until pops are firm.

5. To remove pops from molds, place bottom of pop under warm running water. Press firmly on bottom to release. (Do not twist or pull the pop stick.)

Makes about 6 pops

Pour any extra mixture into small paper cups. Freeze as directed in Tip.

Tip: Three-ounce paper cups can be used in place of the molds. Make the layers as directed or put a single flavor in each cup. Freeze cups about 1 hour, then insert wooden stick (which can be found at craft stores) into the center of each cup. Freeze completely. Peel cup off each pop to serve.

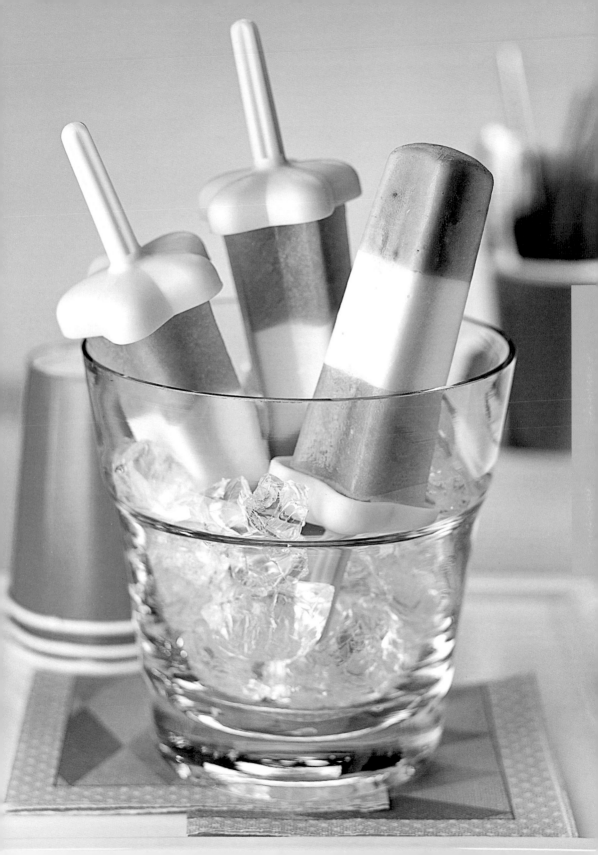

Strawberry Shortcake

2 pounds strawberries, sliced
½ cup sugar, divided
3 cups Gluten-Free All-Purpose Flour Blend (page 108)*
4½ teaspoons baking powder
¾ teaspoon salt
¾ teaspoon xanthan gum
¾ cup (1½ sticks) cold butter, cut into pieces
1 to 1¼ cups half-and-half
1 tablespoon cinnamon-sugar (optional)
Whipped cream

Or use any all-purpose gluten-free flour blend that does not contain xanthan gum.

1. Preheat oven to 400°F. Grease baking sheet or line with parchment paper. Combine strawberries and ¼ cup sugar in medium bowl. Mash slightly to release juices; refrigerate until ready to serve.

2. Combine flour blend, remaining ¼ cup sugar, baking powder, salt and xanthan gum in large bowl. Cut in butter with pastry blender or two knives until mixture resembles coarse crumbs. Gradually add 1 cup half-and-half, stirring with fork until rough dough forms. Add additional half-and-half by tablespoonfuls if needed.

3. Turn dough out onto floured surface. Pat into ¾-inch-thick layer. Cut dough with 2½-inch biscuit cutter; place on prepared baking sheet. Pat remaining dough together and cut out additional biscuits. Brush tops with additional half-and-half and sprinkle with cinnamon-sugar, if desired.

4. Bake 15 to 20 minutes or until golden brown. Transfer to wire rack to cool. Split biscuits; top with strawberry mixture and whipped cream.

Makes 6 to 8 servings

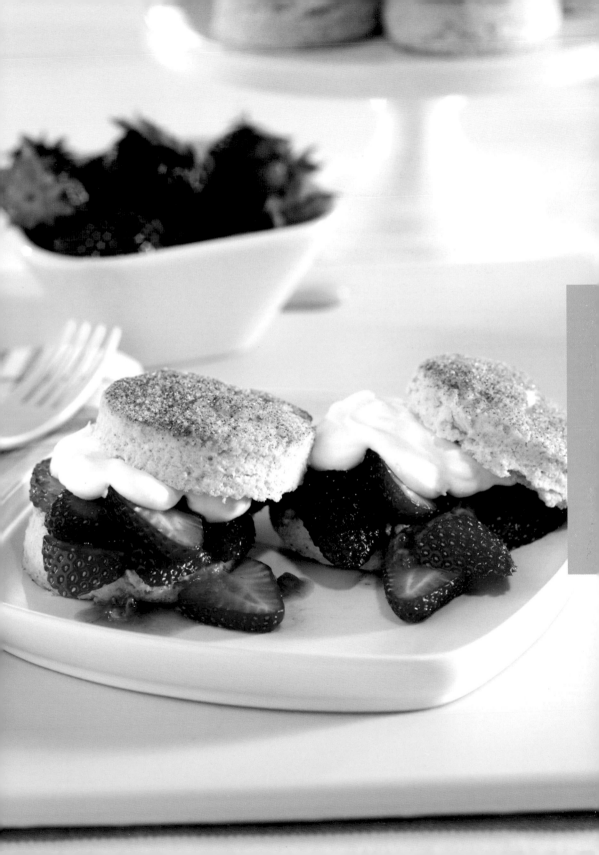

Orange Snickerdoodles

··

½ **cup (1 stick) dairy-free margarine**
1 **cup granulated sugar**
1 **tablespoon grated orange peel**
1 **egg**
½ **teaspoon vanilla**
1½ **cups Gluten-Free All-Purpose Flour Blend (page 108)***
¾ **teaspoon xanthan gum**
½ **teaspoon baking soda**
½ **teaspoon cream of tartar**
¼ **cup orange-colored sugar****

Icing

1 **cup powdered sugar**
2 **tablespoons orange juice**
¼ **teaspoon vanilla**

*Or use any all-purpose gluten-free flour blend that does not contain xanthan gum.
**Or substitute granulated sugar.

1. Beat margarine in large bowl with electric mixer at medium speed for 30 seconds. Add granulated sugar and orange peel; beat 1 minute. Beat in egg and vanilla until well blended. Add flour blend, xanthan gum, baking soda and cream of tartar; beat just until combined. Cover with plastic wrap; refrigerate 1 hour.

2. Preheat oven to 375°F. Line baking sheets with parchment paper.

3. Shape dough into 1-inch balls; roll in orange-colored sugar. Place balls 2 inches apart on prepared baking sheets. Bake 12 to 15 minutes or until edges are light brown. Transfer baking sheets to wire racks; cool 5 minutes.

4. Meanwhile, prepare icing. Whisk powdered sugar, orange juice and vanilla in small bowl until sugar is dissolved. Add more sugar or juice, if needed.

5. Gently loosen cookies from parchment, but leave on sheets. Drizzle icing evenly over warm cookies using whisk or fork. Transfer to wire racks; cool completely. Icing will firm as cookies cool. Store in airtight container.

Makes about 3 dozen cookies

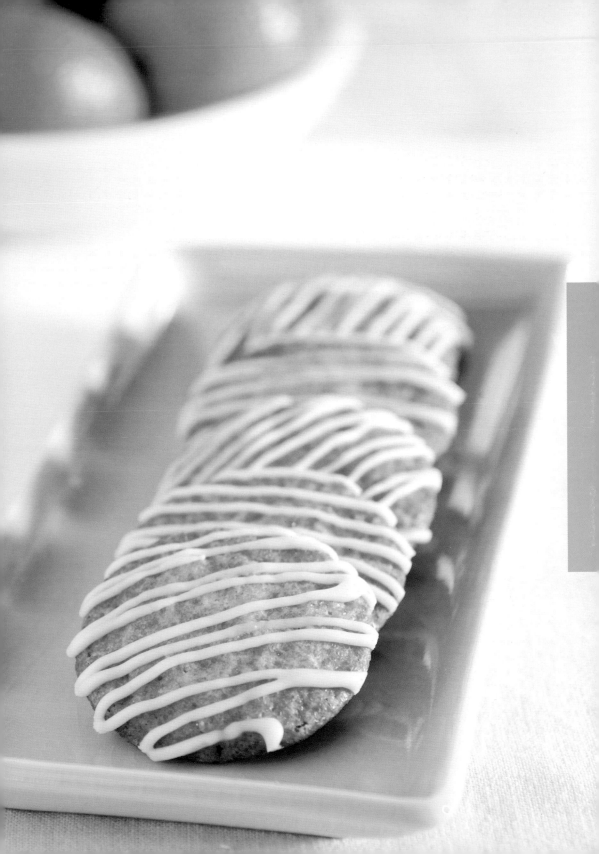

Coconut Milk Ice Cream

2 cans (13½ ounces each) unsweetened coconut milk
½ cup sugar
1 gluten-free dairy-free candy bar, crushed into small pieces

1. Combine coconut milk and sugar in medium saucepan. Cook over medium-low heat, whisking constantly, until smooth and sugar is dissolved. Refrigerate until cold.

2. Process in ice cream maker according to manufacturer's directions adding candy pieces as directed. Transfer to freezer storage container and freeze until firm.

3. To serve, let ice cream soften at room temperature or microwave for 20 to 30 seconds to make scooping easy.   *Makes about 1 quart*

Tip

Many people are sensitive to dairy products as well as gluten. Unsweetened coconut milk makes an excellent substitute for cow's milk. Don't confuse unsweetened coconut milk with the sugary kind (often called coconut cream) that is used to make piña coladas and other tropical drinks.

Safe Kid Stuff

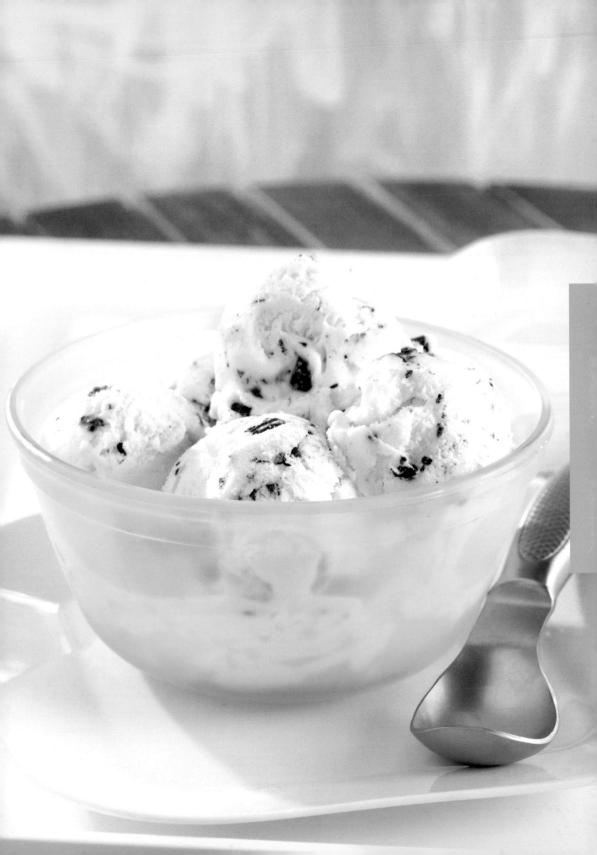

Rocky Road Brownies

½ **cup (1 stick) dairy-free margarine**
½ **cup unsweetened cocoa powder**
1 **cup sugar**
¼ **cup soymilk or other milk**
2 **eggs**
2 **teaspoons vanilla**
⅔ **cup Gluten-Free All-Purpose Flour Blend (page 108)***
½ **teaspoon salt**
½ **teaspoon baking powder**
½ **teaspoon xanthan gum**
1 **cup miniature marshmallows**
1 **cup coarsely chopped walnuts**
1 **cup (6 ounces) semisweet chocolate chips**

*Or use any all-purpose gluten-free flour blend that does not contain xanthan gum.

1. Preheat oven to 350°F. Grease 8-inch square baking pan.

2. Combine margarine and cocoa in large saucepan over low heat, stirring constantly until smooth. Remove from heat; whisk in sugar, soymilk, eggs and vanilla until smooth.

3. Combine flour blend, salt, baking powder and xanthan gum in small bowl. Combine with wet ingredients in saucepan. Spread batter evenly in prepared baking pan.

4. Bake 25 to 35 minutes or until center feels dry. Sprinkle with marshmallows, walnuts and chocolate chips. Bake 3 to 5 minutes or until topping is slightly melted. Cool in pan on wire rack.   *Makes 16 brownies*

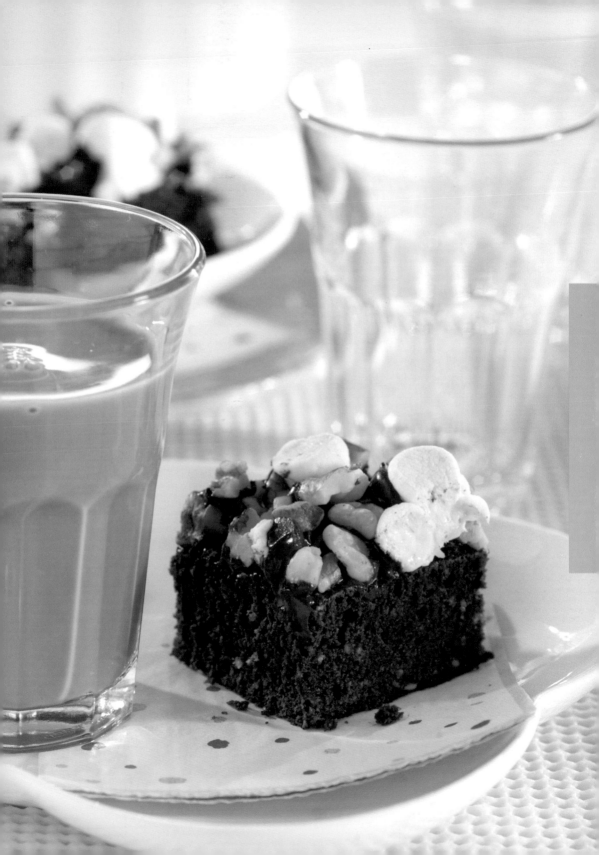

Chocolate Cereal Bars

6 cups gluten-free crisp rice cereal
1 jar (7 ounces) marshmallow creme
1 cup (6 ounces) semisweet chocolate chips
2 tablespoons butter or margarine
1 teaspoon vanilla

1. Grease 13×9-inch baking pan. Place cereal in large heatproof bowl.

2. Melt marshmallow creme, chocolate chips and butter in small heavy saucepan over medium heat, stirring occasionally. Remove from heat; stir in vanilla.

3. Pour chocolate mixture over cereal; stir until blended. Press into prepared pan. Cool before cutting into squares.   *Makes 2 dozen bars*

Flourless Peanut Butter Chocolate Chippers

1 cup packed light brown sugar
1 cup creamy or chunky peanut butter*
1 egg
½ cup chocolate chips
Granulated sugar

*Do not use "natural" peanut butter.

1. Preheat oven to 350°F.

2. Beat brown sugar, peanut butter and egg in medium bowl with electric mixer at medium speed until well blended.

3. Shape dough into 1½-inch balls; place 2 inches apart on ungreased cookie sheets. Dip fork into granulated sugar; flatten each ball to ½-inch thickness, crisscrossing with fork. Press 3 to 4 chocolate chips on top of each cookie.

4. Bake 12 minutes or just until set. Cool on cookie sheets 2 minutes. Remove to wire racks; cool completely.   *Makes 1½ dozen cookies*

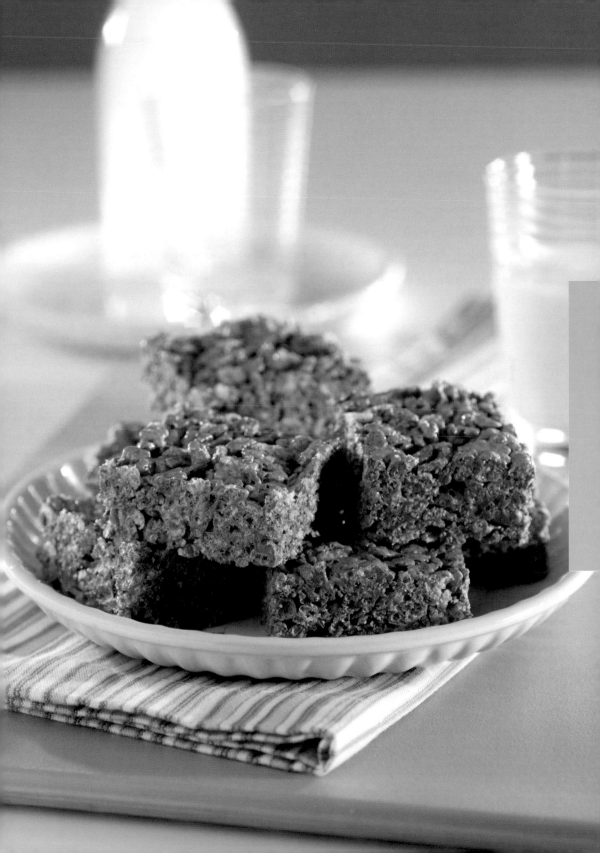

Cookie Heaven

Homemade Coconut Meringues

3 **egg whites**
¼ **teaspoon cream of tartar**
⅛ **teaspoon salt**
¾ **cup sugar**
2¼ **cups flaked coconut, toasted***
1 **teaspoon vanilla**

*To toast coconut, spread evenly on baking sheet. Bake in preheated 350°F oven 5 to 7 minutes or until light golden brown, stirring occasionally. Cool before using.

1. Preheat oven to 300°F. Line cookie sheets with parchment paper or foil.

2. Beat egg whites, cream of tartar and salt in large bowl with electric mixer at high speed until soft peaks form. Beat in sugar, 1 tablespoon at a time, until egg whites are stiff and shiny. Fold in coconut and vanilla. Drop dough by tablespoonfuls 2 inches apart onto prepared cookie sheets; flatten slightly.

3. Bake 18 to 22 minutes or until golden brown. Cool on cookie sheets 1 minute; transfer to wire racks to cool completely. Store in airtight container.

Makes 2 dozen cookies

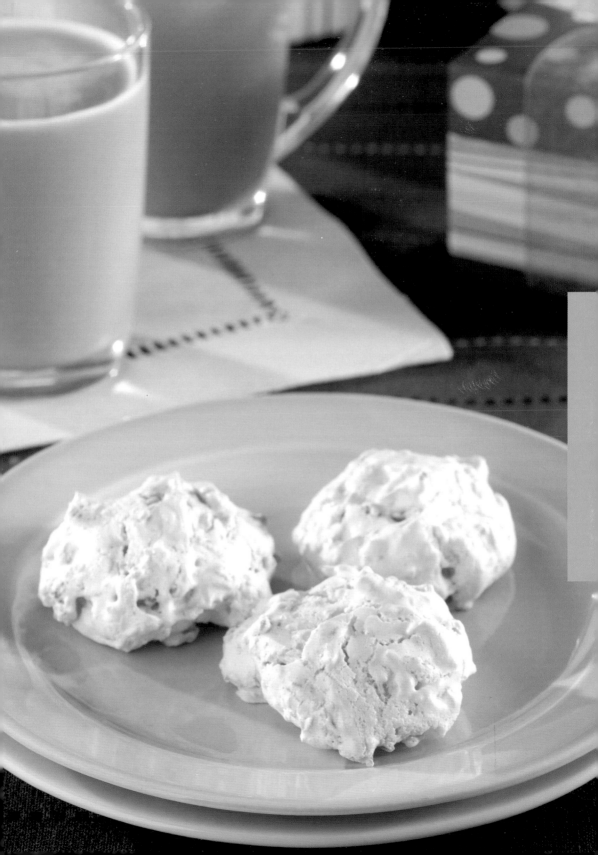

Flourless Peanut Butter Cookies

1 cup packed light brown sugar
1 cup creamy peanut butter
1 egg, lightly beaten
½ cup semisweet chocolate chips, melted

1. Preheat oven to 350°F. Beat brown sugar, peanut butter and egg in medium bowl with electric mixer until blended and smooth.

2. Shape dough into 24 balls; place 2 inches apart on ungreased cookie sheets. Flatten slightly with fork.

3. Bake 10 to 12 minutes or until set. Remove to wire racks; cool completely. Drizzle with chocolate. *Makes 2 dozen cookies*

Variation: Press a milk chocolate star or milk chocolate kiss into each cookie ball before baking instead of drizzling with melted chocolate.

Flourless Almond Cookies

1 cup sugar
1 cup almond butter
1 egg, lightly beaten

1. Preheat oven to 350°F. Beat sugar, almond butter and egg in medium bowl with electric mixer until blended and smooth.

2. Shape dough into 24 balls; place 2 inches apart on ungreased cookie sheets. Flatten slightly with fork.

3. Bake 10 to 12 minutes or until set. Transfer to wire racks to cool.

Makes 2 dozen cookies

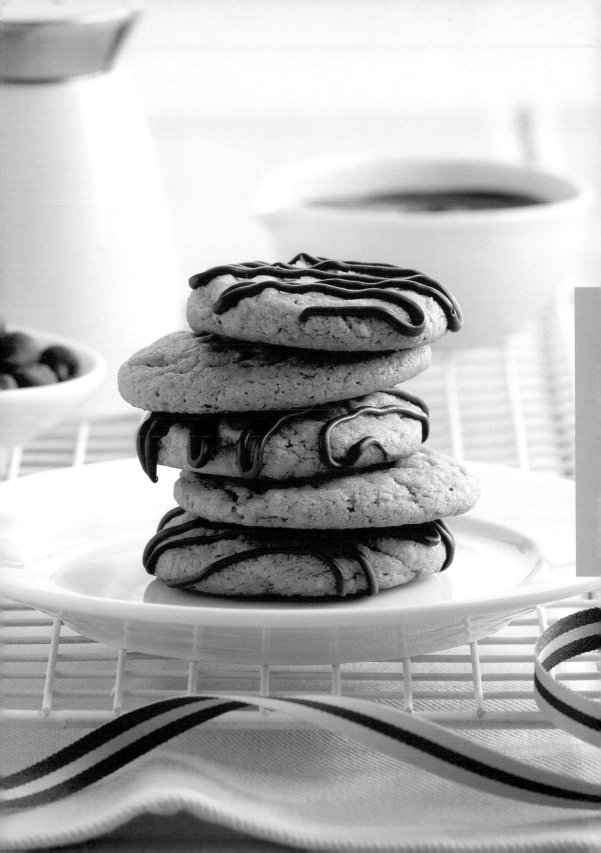

Caramel Chocolate Chunk Blondies

1½ **cups Gluten-Free All-Purpose Flour Blend (page 108)***

1 **teaspoon baking powder**

½ **teaspoon xanthan gum**

½ **teaspoon salt**

¾ **cup granulated sugar**

¾ **cup packed brown sugar**

½ **cup (1 stick) dairy-free margarine**

2 **eggs**

1½ **teaspoons vanilla**

1½ **cups semisweet chocolate chunks**

⅓ **cup caramel ice cream topping**

Or use any all-purpose gluten-free flour blend that does not contain xanthan gum.

1. Preheat oven to 350°F. Spray 13×9-inch baking pan with nonstick cooking spray.

2. Combine flour blend, baking powder, xanthan gum and salt in medium bowl. Beat granulated sugar, brown sugar and margarine in large bowl with electric mixer at medium speed until smooth and creamy. Beat in eggs and vanilla until well blended. Add flour mixture; beat at low speed until blended. Stir in chocolate chunks.

3. Spread batter evenly in prepared pan. Drop spoonfuls of caramel topping over batter; swirl into batter with knife.

4. Bake 25 minutes or until golden brown. Cool completely in pan on wire rack.

Makes about 2½ dozen blondies

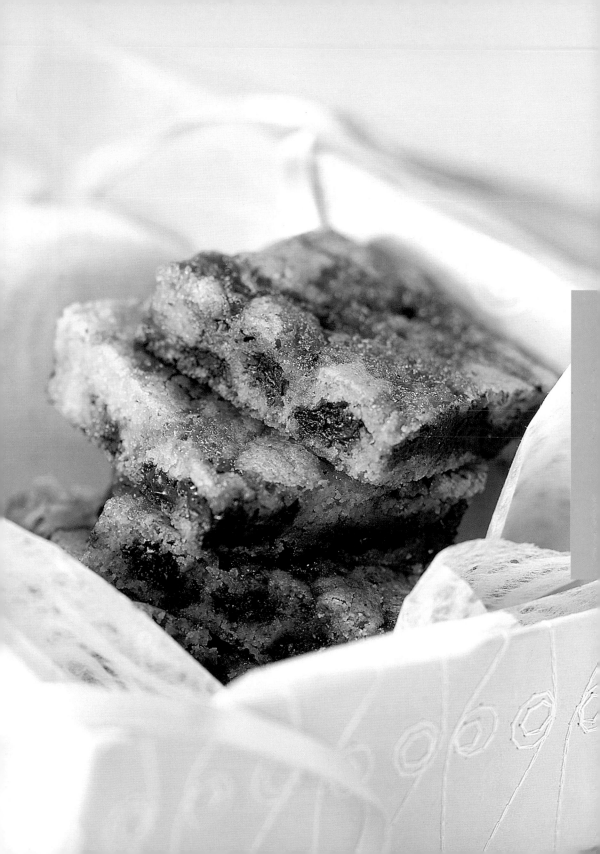

Raisin-Coconut Cookies

1¾ cups **Gluten-Free All-Purpose Flour Blend (page 108)***

  2 teaspoons **baking powder**

  ½ teaspoon **xanthan gum**

  ½ teaspoon **salt**

  1 cup **(2 sticks) dairy-free margarine**

  ½ cup **granulated sugar**

  ½ cup **packed brown sugar**

  1 **egg**

  1 teaspoon **vanilla**

  2 cups **flaked coconut**

1½ cups **raisins**

Or use any all-purpose gluten-free flour blend that does not contain xanthan gum.

1. Preheat oven to 350°F. Line cookie sheets with parchment paper.

2. Whisk flour blend, baking powder, xanthan gum and salt in medium bowl.

3. Beat margarine, granulated sugar and brown sugar in large bowl with electric mixer at medium speed about 2 minutes or until well blended. Beat in egg and vanilla. Add flour mixture; beat at low speed about 30 seconds or just until combined. Stir in coconut and raisins. Drop dough by rounded tablespoonfuls 2 inches apart onto prepared cookie sheets.

4. Bake 10 to 12 minutes or until brown around edges (centers will be light). Remove to wire racks; cool completely. *Makes about 4 dozen cookies*

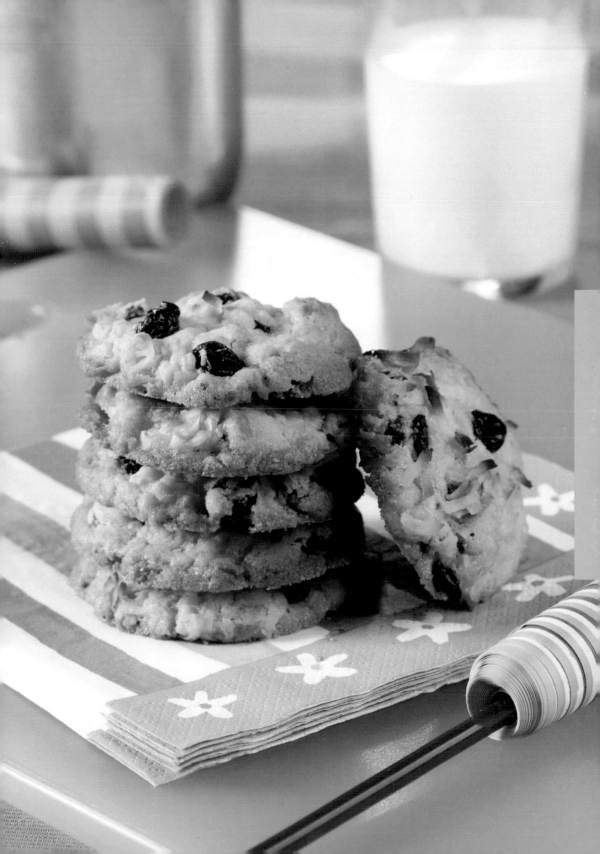

Crispy Toffee Cookies

½ cup rice flour
½ cup dry roasted peanuts
⅛ teaspoon salt
½ cup packed brown sugar
⅓ cup dairy-free margarine
¼ cup light corn syrup
1 teaspoon vanilla
¼ cup chocolate chips, melted

1. Preheat oven to 375°F. Line two cookie sheets with parchment paper.

2. Combine rice flour, peanuts and salt in food processor; process until mixture resembles coarse crumbs.

3. Combine brown sugar, margarine and corn syrup in medium saucepan; bring to a full boil over medium heat, stirring frequently. Remove from heat; stir in peanut mixture and vanilla until well blended. Return to low heat to keep batter warm and pliable. Spoon 6 rounded ½ teaspoonfuls of batter 3 inches apart on one prepared cookie sheet.

4. Bake exactly 4 minutes. While cookies are baking, spoon batter on second cookie sheet. When cookies have baked 4 minutes, immediately remove from oven. (Cookies will have very light color and will appear not to be completely baked.) Remove parchment paper and cookies to wire rack to cool completely.

5. While second batch of cookies is baking, line first cookie sheet with new sheet of parchment paper; continue to prepare and bake cookies in batches of six. (Sheets of parchment paper can be reused after cookies are removed.)

6. Peel cookies from parchment paper; remove to wire rack. Drizzle melted chocolate over cookies; let stand until set. Store cookies in airtight container with parchment paper or waxed paper between layers to prevent cookies from sticking together. *Makes about 4 dozen cookies*

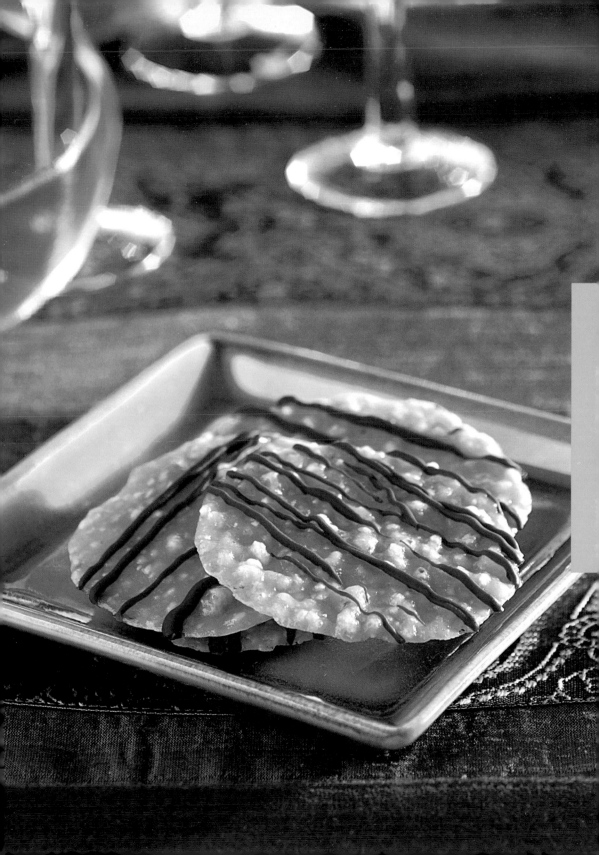

Choco-Coco Pecan Crisps

1 cup packed light brown sugar

½ cup (1 stick) butter, softened

1 egg

1 teaspoon vanilla

1½ cups Gluten-Free All-Purpose Flour Blend (page 108)*

1 cup chopped pecans

⅓ cup unsweetened cocoa powder

½ teaspoon baking soda

½ teaspoon xanthan gum

1 cup flaked coconut

*Or use any all-purpose gluten-free flour blend that does not contain xanthan gum.

1. Beat brown sugar and butter in large bowl with electric mixer at medium speed until light and fluffy. Beat in egg and vanilla. Combine flour blend, pecans, cocoa, baking soda and xanthan gum in small bowl until well blended. Add to butter mixture, blending until stiff dough is formed.

2. Sprinkle coconut on work surface. Divide dough into 4 pieces. Shape each piece into log about 1½ inches in diameter; roll in coconut until thickly coated. Wrap in plastic wrap; refrigerate until firm, at least 1 hour or up to 2 weeks. (For longer storage, freeze up to 6 weeks.)

3. Preheat oven to 350°F. Cut rolls into ⅛-inch-thick slices. Place 2 inches apart on ungreased cookie sheets. Bake 10 to 13 minutes or until firm. Remove to wire racks to cool.   *Makes about 6 dozen cookies*

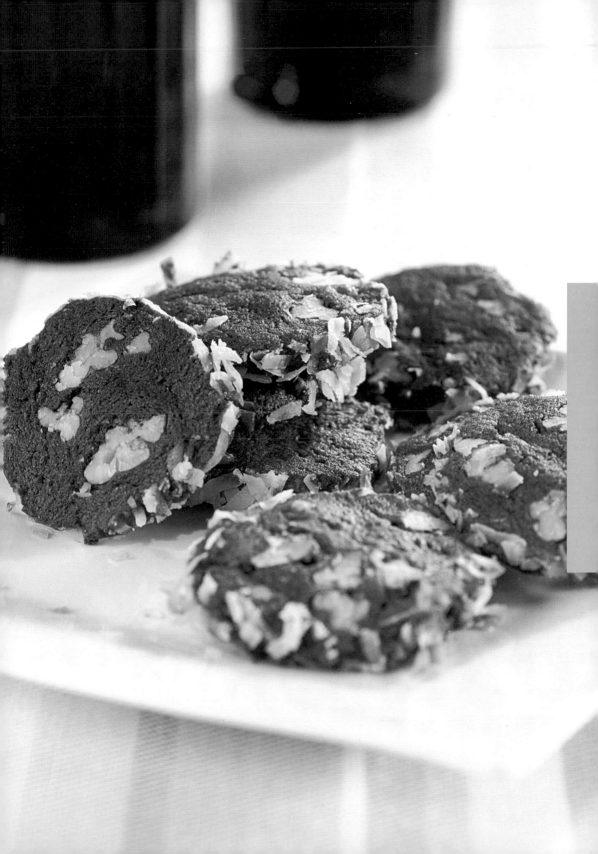

Cranberry Chocolate Chip Cereal Squares

6½ cups gluten-free corn or rice cereal squares
1 package (6 ounces) dried cranberries (about 1⅓ cups)
½ cup (1 stick) dairy-free margarine
1 bag (about 10 ounces) miniature marshmallows
1 cup semisweet chocolate chips

1. Line 13×9-inch pan with foil; spray foil with nonstick cooking spray.

2. Place 2 cups cereal in large bowl. Coarsely crush with back of spoon or hands. Stir in cranberries.

3. Melt margarine in large saucepan over low heat. Add marshmallows; stir constantly until melted and smooth. Remove from heat; stir in remaining 4½ cups whole cereal and crushed cereal mixture until well blended. Stir in chocolate chips.

4. Press mixture into prepared pan. Cover and refrigerate 30 minutes or until firm. Remove from pan using foil; cut into squares.

Makes about 30 squares

Tip

Marshmallows are thickened with cornstarch and gelatin and almost always gluten-free. Now there are many gluten-free cereals in the supermarket as well, so it's easy to whip up a delicious batch of crispy cereal treats.

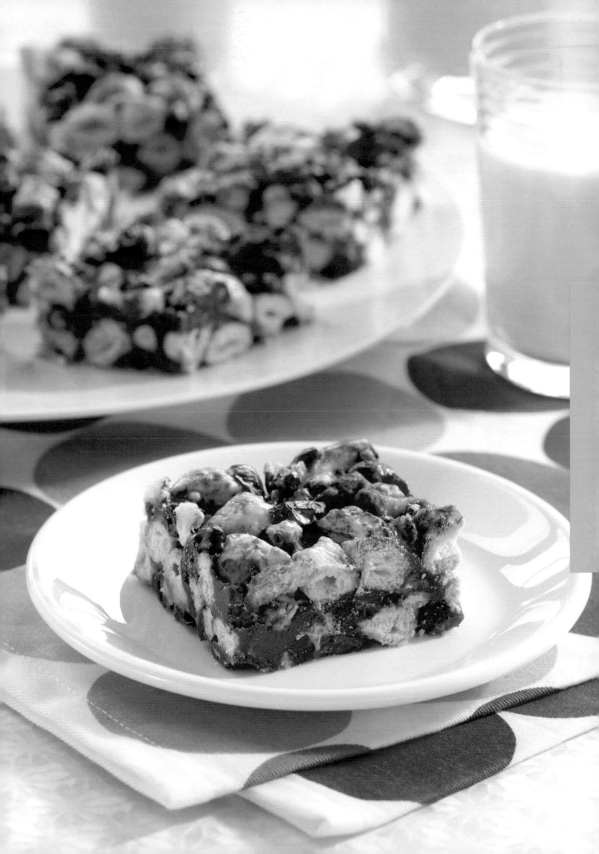

Almond Crescents

1 cup (2 sticks) butter, softened
⅓ cup granulated sugar
1¾ cups Gluten-Free All-Purpose Flour Blend (page 108)*
¼ cup cornstarch
1 teaspoon vanilla
½ teaspoon xanthan gum
1½ cups ground toasted almonds (see Tip)**
Chocolate Glaze (recipe follows)

Or use any all-purpose gluten-free flour blend that does not contain xanthan gum.

**To toast almonds, spread in single layer on baking sheet. Bake in preheated 350°F oven 8 to 10 minutes or until golden brown, stirring frequently.*

1. Preheat oven to 325°F. Beat butter and granulated sugar in large bowl with electric mixer at medium speed until creamy. Mix in flour blend, cornstarch, vanilla and xanthan gum. Stir in ground almonds. Shape tablespoonfuls of dough into crescents. Place 2 inches apart on ungreased cookie sheets.

2. Bake 22 to 25 minutes or until light brown. Cool on cookie sheets 1 minute. Remove to wire racks; cool completely. Prepare Chocolate Glaze; drizzle over cookies. Let stand until chocolate is set; store in airtight container.

Makes about 3 dozen cookies

Chocolate Glaze: Place ½ cup semisweet chocolate chips and 1 tablespoon butter in small resealable food storage bag. Place bag in bowl of hot water for 2 to 3 minutes or until chocolate is softened. Knead until chocolate mixture is smooth. Cut off very tiny corner of bag. Drizzle over cookies.

Tip

To grind almonds, place them in a food processor. Process using on/off pulses until finely ground. Do not overprocess or you will end up with almond butter. Adding a tablespoon or two of powdered sugar to the almonds can help prevent this.

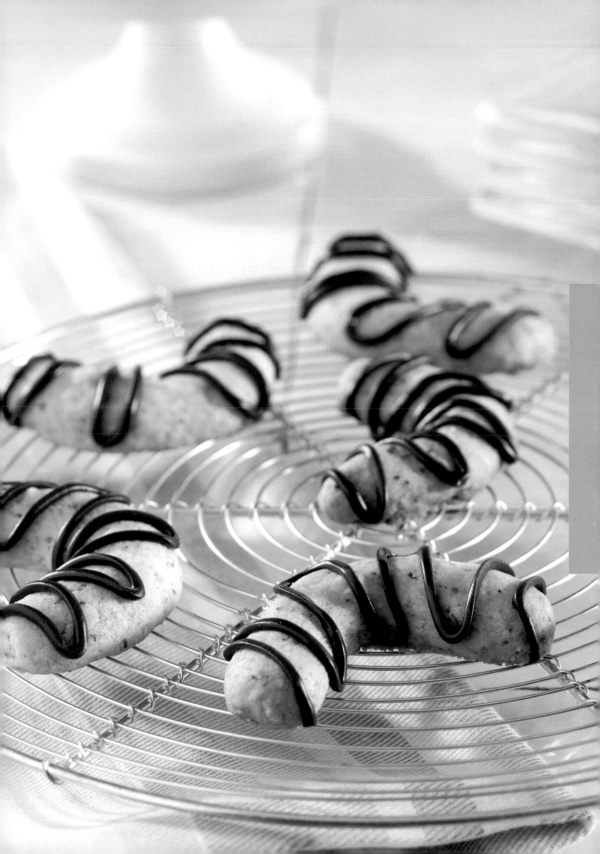

Gluten-Free Lemon Bars

....

1 cup Gluten-Free All-Purpose Flour Blend (page 108)*
1 cup macadamia nuts or slivered almonds
½ cup (1 stick) cold butter, cut into pieces
½ cup powdered sugar
1 tablespoon plus 1 teaspoon grated lemon peel, divided
½ teaspoon salt
1 cup granulated sugar
3 eggs
⅓ cup lemon juice
Additional powdered sugar for dusting
Or use any all-purpose gluten-free flour blend that does not contain xanthan gum.

1. Preheat oven to 350°F. Spray 9-inch square baking pan with nonstick cooking spray.

2. Place flour blend, nuts, butter, powdered sugar, 1 teaspoon lemon peel and salt in food processor. Process until mixture forms fine crumbs. Press mixture onto bottom of prepared pan. Bake 15 minutes or until light golden brown.

3. Beat granulated sugar, eggs, lemon juice and remaining 1 tablespoon lemon peel in large bowl with electric mixer at medium speed until blended.

4. Pour mixture evenly over warm crust. Bake 18 to 20 minutes or until center is set and edges are golden brown. Cool completely in pan on wire rack. Dust with additional powdered sugar. Store tightly covered at room temperature.

Makes 1½ dozen bars

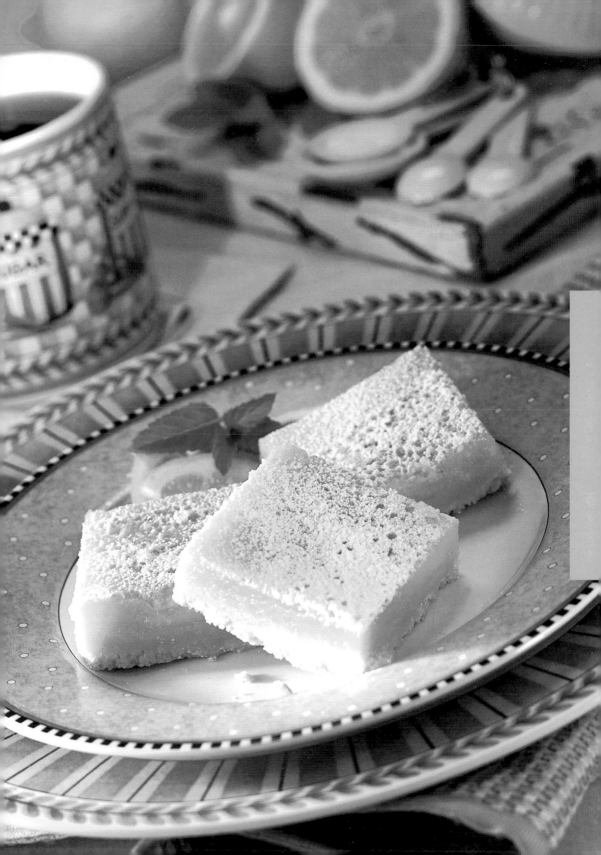

Holiday Cut-Out Cookies

¾ **cup granulated sugar**
½ **cup shortening**
1 **egg**
2 **cups Gluten-Free All-Purpose Flour Blend (page 108)***
1 **teaspoon xanthan gum**
1 **teaspoon ground cinnamon**
½ **teaspoon salt**
½ **teaspoon baking powder**
2 **teaspoons vanilla**
2 **to 3 tablespoons soymilk or other milk**
  Fluffy White Frosting (page 196)
  Food coloring (optional)
  Colored sugar

Or use any all-purpose gluten-free flour blend that does not contain xanthan gum.

1. Beat granulated sugar and shortening in large bowl with electric mixer 2 minutes or until light and fluffy. Beat in egg.

2. Whisk flour blend, xanthan gum, cinnamon, salt and baking powder in medium bowl. Gradually beat into sugar mixture. Beat in vanilla and 2 tablespoons soymilk to make soft dough. Add additional milk by teaspoonfuls if dough is too dry. Divide dough in half; pat into discs. Wrap and refrigerate 15 minutes.

3. Preheat oven to 350°F. Line baking sheets with parchment paper.

4. Roll out each half of dough between sheets of waxed paper until ¼ inch thick. Cut out cookies and transfer to prepared baking sheets. Bake 8 to 10 minutes or until edges begin to brown. Cool completely on wire racks. Meanwhile, prepare Fluffy White Frosting and tint with food coloring, if desired. Frost cookies and sprinkle with colored sugar.

Makes about 2 dozen cookies

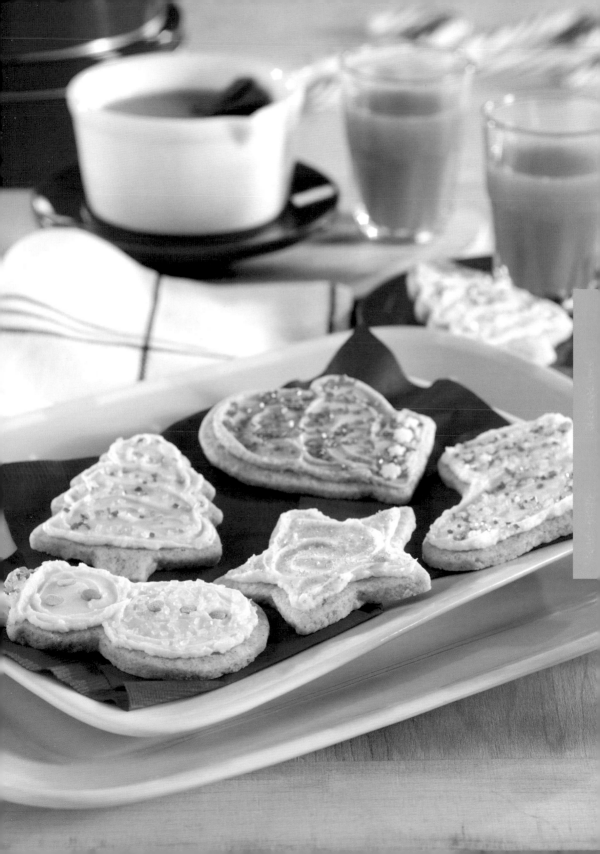

Let's Celebrate

Coconut Panna Cotta

3 tablespoons water
1 envelope (2½ teaspoons) unflavored gelatin
1 can (about 13 ounces) unsweetened coconut milk
½ cup sugar
½ teaspoon vanilla
4 tablespoons toasted flaked coconut
2 slices (½ inch thick) fresh pineapple, cut into pieces

1. Place water in small bowl and sprinkle with gelatin; set aside.

2. Heat coconut milk, sugar and vanilla in medium saucepan over medium heat. Cook and stir until sugar is dissolved and mixture is smooth. *Do not boil.* Add gelatin mixture; stir until gelatin is completely dissolved.

3. Pour mixture evenly into four 5-ounce custard cups. Refrigerate about 3 hours or until set.

4. To unmold, run knife around outside edges of cups; place cups in hot water about 30 seconds. Place serving plate over cup; invert and shake until panna cotta drops onto plate. Serve with toasted coconut and pineapple. Refrigerate leftovers.

Makes 4 servings

Note: Panna cotta is best eaten within 2 days.

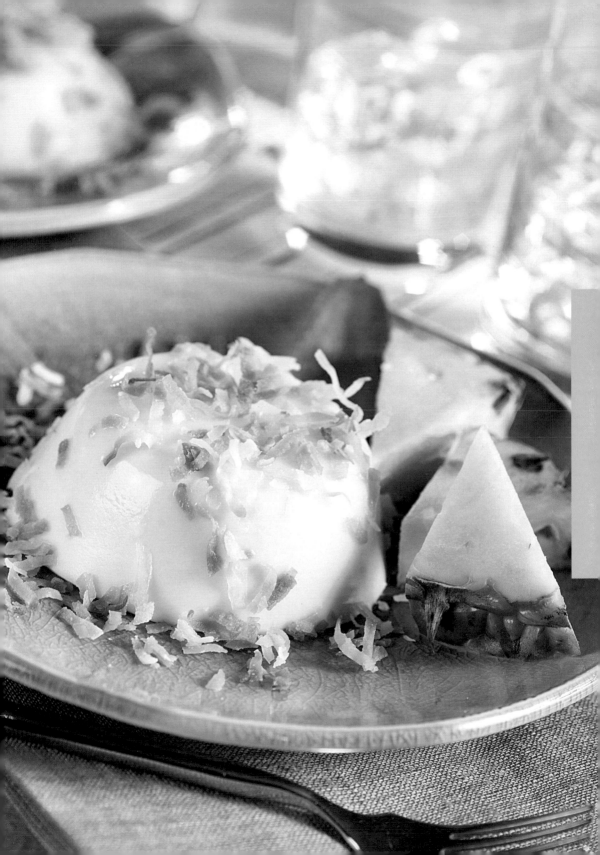

Yellow Layer Cake

2 cups Gluten-Free All-Purpose Flour Blend (page 108),* plus additional for pans

1¼ teaspoons baking powder

½ teaspoon salt

½ teaspoon xanthan gum

1¼ cups sugar

1 cup (2 sticks) dairy-free margarine

4 eggs

2 teaspoons vanilla

¼ cup soymilk or other milk

Dark Chocolate Frosting (page 188)

Or use any all-purpose gluten-free flour blend that does not contain xanthan gum.

1. Preheat oven to 350°F. Spray two 9-inch round cake pans with nonstick cooking spray. Line bottoms with parchment paper or dust with flour blend.

2. Combine flour blend, baking powder, salt and xanthan gum in medium bowl.

3. Beat sugar and margarine in large bowl with electric mixer at medium speed 8 minutes or until light and fluffy. Add eggs, one at a time, beating well after each addition. Beat in vanilla.

4. Add flour mixture and soymilk alternately to sugar mixture, beating at low speed and scraping side and bottom of bowl occasionally. Beat at medium speed 2 minutes.

5. Divide batter between prepared pans. Tap bottoms of pans on counter to even out batter. Bake 35 to 40 minutes or until toothpick inserted into centers comes out clean.

6. Cool in pans on wire rack 5 minutes. Remove from pans and cool completely.

7. Meanwhile, prepare Dark Chocolate Frosting. Frost cake.

Makes 10 servings

continued on page 188

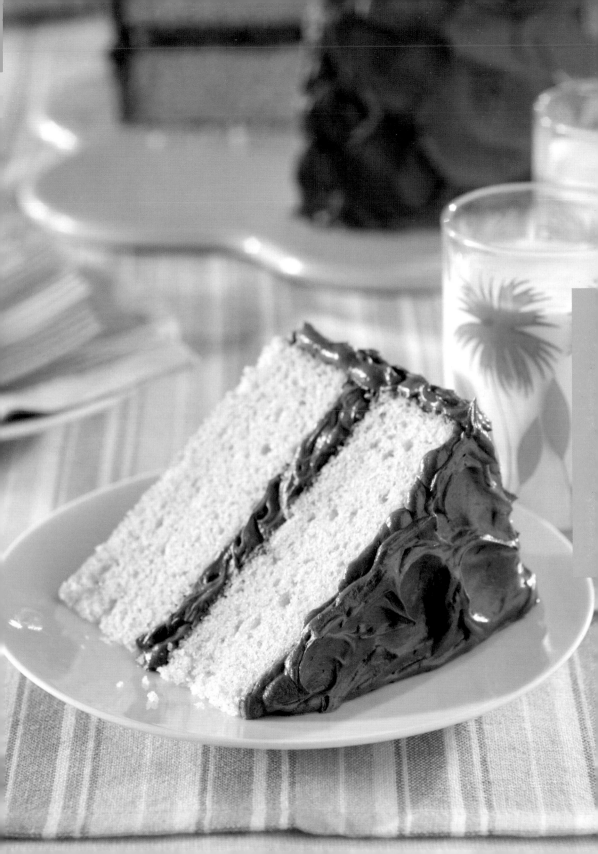

Dark Chocolate Frosting

··

  1 cup (2 sticks) dairy-free margarine
  3 cups sifted powdered sugar
  7 ounces semisweet chocolate, melted
  ⅓ cup unsweetened cocoa powder
  ⅔ to 1 cup soy creamer
1½ teaspoons vanilla

Beat margarine in medium bowl with electric mixer at medium speed until light and fluffy. Gradually beat in powdered sugar, alternating with melted chocolate and cocoa. Beat in soy creamer by tablespoonfuls until spreadable. Beat in vanilla.

Praline Pumpkin Pie

··

1½ cups solid-pack pumpkin
  ½ cup sugar
  ½ teaspoon salt
  1 teaspoon ground cinnamon
  ½ teaspoon ground ginger
  ½ teaspoon ground cloves
1½ cups whipping cream
  2 eggs
  4 tablespoons flaked coconut, divided
  4 tablespoons chopped pecans, divided

1. Preheat oven to 425°F. Stir together pumpkin, sugar, salt and spices in medium bowl. Stir in cream and eggs until well blended.

2. Sprinkle 2 tablespoons coconut and 2 tablespoons pecans in 9-inch pie pan. Pour in pumpkin mixture. Sprinkle with remaining coconut and pecans. Bake 15 minutes. *Reduce oven temperature to 350°F.* Bake 45 minutes or until knife inserted into center comes out clean.
        Makes 8 servings

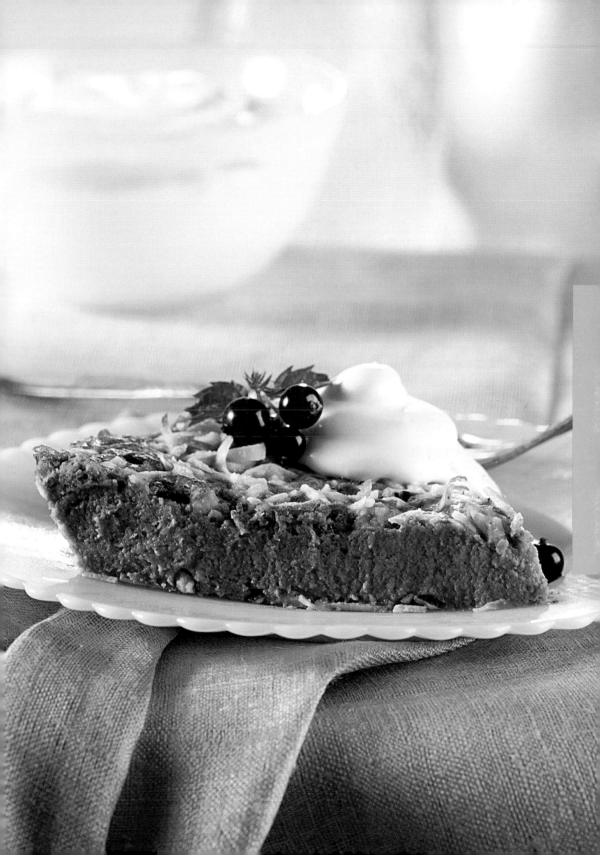

Cherry Pink Cupcakes

1 jar (6 ounces) maraschino cherries

1 cup granulated sugar

2 eggs

1¼ cups Gluten-Free All-Purpose Flour Blend (page 108)*

1½ teaspoons baking powder

½ teaspoon salt

½ teaspoon xanthan gum

½ cup vegetable oil

½ cup soymilk or other milk

1 teaspoon vanilla

Cherry Pink Frosting (recipe follows)

Stemmed cherries (optional)

Or use any all-purpose gluten-free flour blend that does not contain xanthan gum.

1. Preheat oven to 350°F. Line 12 standard (2½-inch) muffin cups with paper baking cups. Drain cherries reserving juice for Cherry Pink Frosting. Chop cherries and squeeze out excess moisture. Spread cherries on paper towels to drain. Set aside.

2. Beat sugar and eggs in large bowl with electric mixer at medium speed until light and fluffy. Combine flour blend, baking powder, salt and xanthan gum in medium bowl. Add dry ingredients to sugar mixture; beat until combined.

3. Add oil, soymilk and vanilla; beat 1 minute or until smooth. Stir in chopped cherries.

4. Pour batter into prepared muffin cups, filling three-fourths full. Bake 20 minutes or until lightly browned and centers spring back when gently touched. Cool in pan on wire rack 5 minutes. Remove from pan and cool completely. Meanwhile, prepare Cherry Pink Frosting; frost cupcakes and garnish with cherries. *Makes 12 cupcakes*

Cherry Pink Frosting: Beat ½ cup (1 stick) dairy-free margarine in medium bowl with electric mixer at medium speed until light and fluffy. Add 1 cup powdered sugar; beat until blended. Add 4 teaspoons of reserved cherry juice and 1 cup powdered sugar; beat until smooth. Add drops of red food coloring for a darker pink. Add additional powdered sugar until frosting is spreadable.

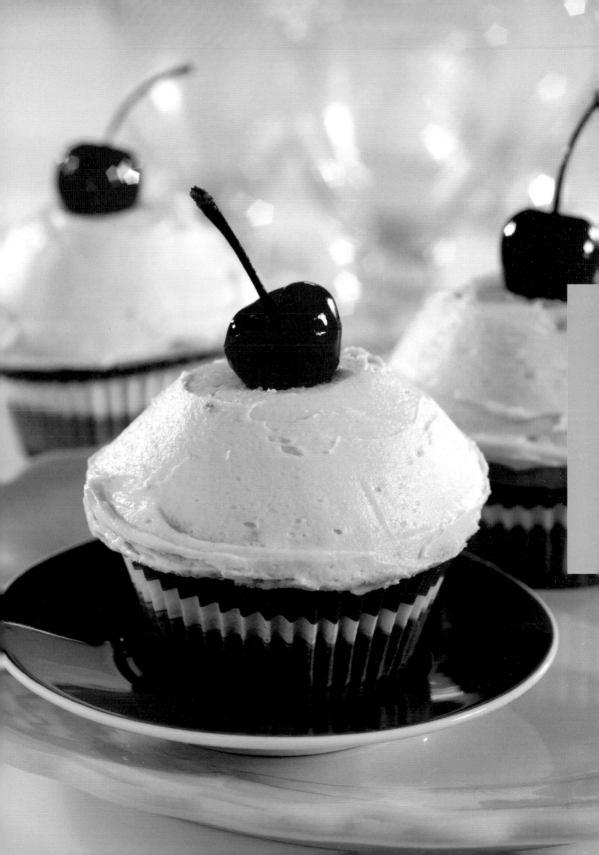

Chocolate Peppermint Macaroons

4 ounces bittersweet chocolate, chopped (½ cup)

2 squares (1 ounce each) unsweetened baking chocolate

2 egg whites, at room temperature

⅛ teaspoon salt

½ cup sugar

½ teaspoon peppermint extract

2¾ cups flaked coconut

½ cup finely crushed peppermint candies*

*About 18 peppermint candies will yield ½ cup finely crushed peppermints. To crush, place unwrapped candy in a heavy-duty resealable food storage bag. Loosely seal the bag, leaving an opening for air to escape. Crush with a rolling pin, meat mallet or the bottom of a heavy skillet.

1. Line cookie sheets with parchment paper or lightly grease.

2. Place bittersweet and unsweetened chocolate in medium microwavable bowl. Microwave on HIGH at 30-second intervals, stirring between each interval, until melted and smooth.** Let stand 15 minutes.

3. Preheat oven to 325°F. Beat egg whites and salt in large bowl with electric mixer at high speed until soft peaks form. Gradually add sugar, beating until stiff peaks form. Add chocolate; beat at low speed just until blended. Stir in peppermint extract. Fold in coconut until blended.

4. Shape level tablespoonfuls into 1-inch balls; place 2 inches apart on prepared cookie sheets. Make small indentation in center. Sprinkle crushed candy into indentations. Bake 12 minutes or until outside is crisp and inside is moist and chewy. Remove to wire racks; cool completely.

Makes 2 dozen macaroons

**Or place chocolate in top of double boiler over simmering water. Stir constantly until melted and smooth. Remove from heat immediately. Avoid getting any water in the chocolate or it will become brittle and hard.

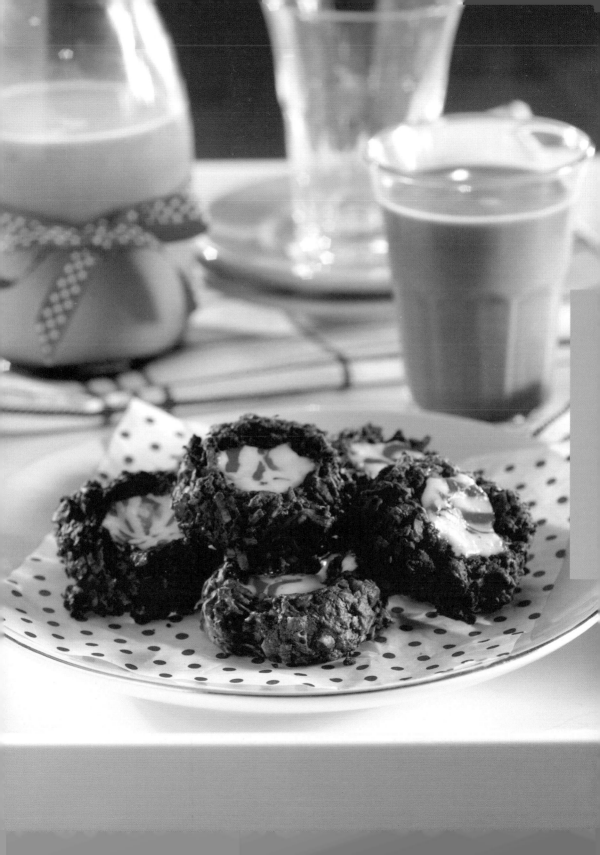

Choco-Berry Cake

2 cups Gluten-Free All-Purpose Flour Blend (page 108),* plus additional
   for pans
1 cup unsweetened cocoa powder
1 cup granulated sugar
1 cup packed brown sugar
2 teaspoons baking powder
1 teaspoon baking soda
1 teaspoon xanthan gum
1 teaspoon espresso powder (optional)
½ teaspoon salt
1½ cups soymilk or other milk
½ cup vegetable oil
2 eggs
2 teaspoons vanilla
1 cup semisweet chocolate chips
   Fluffy White Frosting (page 196)
1 pint strawberries, sliced (about 2 cups), plus additional for garnish

Or use any all-purpose gluten-free flour blend that does not contain xanthan gum.

1. Preheat oven to 350°F. Grease and flour two 9-inch round cake pans.

2. Combine flour blend, cocoa, granulated sugar, brown sugar, baking powder, baking soda, xanthan gum, espresso powder, if desired, and salt in large bowl. Mix until well combined.

3. Mix soymilk, oil, eggs and vanilla in medium bowl. Add to dry ingredients; stir until well blended. Stir in chocolate chips.

4. Divide batter between prepared pans. Bake on center rack of oven 35 to 45 minutes or until toothpick inserted into centers comes out clean.

5. Cool in pans on wire rack 5 minutes; remove from pans and cool completely. Meanwhile, prepare Fluffy White Frosting.

6. Place one layer on serving plate. Spread with thin layer of frosting. Arrange sliced strawberries over frosting. Top with second layer. Frost and garnish with additional strawberries.

Makes 10 servings

continued on page 196

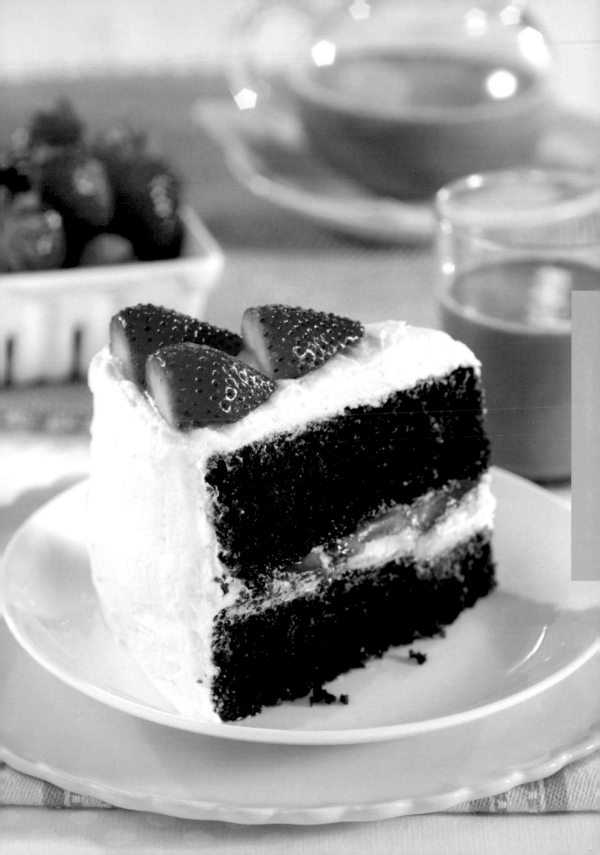

Choco-Berry Cake, continued

Fluffy White Frosting: Beat 1½ cups (3 sticks) dairy-free margarine and 1½ teaspoons vanilla in medium bowl with electric mixer until light and fluffy. Add 3 cups powdered sugar and ½ teaspoon salt; beat until blended. Beat in 3 tablespoons vanilla-flavor soy creamer. Beat in additional 3 cups powdered sugar and additional creamer by tablespoonfuls until frosting is spreadable.

Hidden Pumpkin Pies

1½ **cups solid-pack pumpkin**
1 **cup evaporated milk**
2 **eggs**
¼ **cup sugar**
1¼ **teaspoons vanilla, divided**
1 **teaspoon pumpkin pie spice**
3 **egg whites**
¼ **teaspoon cream of tartar**
⅓ **cup honey**

1. Preheat oven to 350°F. Combine pumpkin, evaporated milk, eggs, sugar, 1 teaspoon vanilla and pumpkin pie spice in large bowl; mix well. Pour into six 6-ounce custard cups or soufflé dishes. Place in shallow baking dish or pan. Pour boiling water around custard cups to depth of 1 inch. Bake 25 minutes or until set.

2. Meanwhile, beat egg whites, cream of tartar and remaining ¼ teaspoon vanilla in medium bowl with electric mixer at high speed until soft peaks form. Gradually add honey, beating until stiff peaks form.

3. Spread egg white mixture over hot pumpkin pies. Bake 8 to 12 minutes or until tops of pies are golden brown. Let stand 10 minutes. Serve warm.

Makes 6 servings

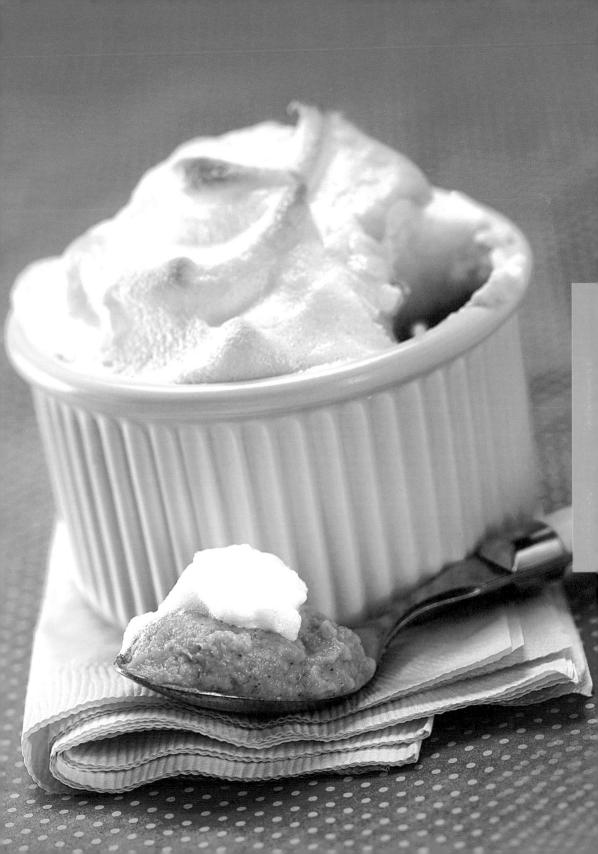

Raspberry Clafouti

3 eggs*
⅓ cup sugar
1 cup half-and-half
2 tablespoons butter, melted and slightly cooled
½ teaspoon vanilla
⅔ cup almond flour
Pinch salt
2 containers (6 ounces each) fresh raspberries

Use the highest quality eggs possible since the flavor of this dessert depends upon them.

1. Preheat oven to 325°F. Generously butter 9-inch ceramic tart pan or pie plate.

2. Beat eggs and sugar in large bowl with electric mixer at medium speed 3 to 5 minutes or until slightly thickened. Add half-and-half, butter and vanilla; whisk to combine. Gradually whisk in almond flour and salt. Pour enough batter into prepared pan to just cover bottom. Bake 10 minutes or until batter firms.

3. Remove from oven and scatter raspberries over baked batter. Stir remaining batter and pour over raspberries.

4. Bake 40 to 45 minutes or until clafouti is set in center and top is golden. Cool on wire rack to room temperature before serving. Refrigerate leftovers.

Makes 8 to 10 servings

Tip

Clafouti is a rustic French dessert that is made by topping fresh fruit with a custard-like batter and baking. The most famous and traditional clafouti is made with cherries, but berries, plums, peaches and pears are also used.

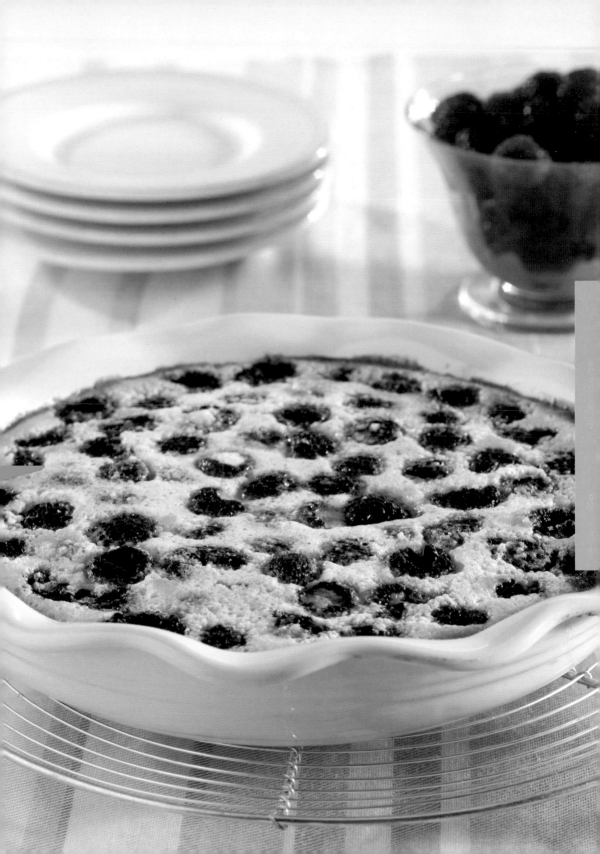

Allergy-Free Birthday Cake

3 cups Gluten-Free All-Purpose Flour Blend (page 108),* plus additional for pans

2 cups sugar

6 tablespoons unsweetened cocoa powder

2 teaspoons baking soda

2 teaspoons xanthan gum

1 teaspoon salt

2 cups chocolate soymilk

½ cup plus 2 tablespoons vegetable oil

2 tablespoons cider vinegar

1 teaspoon vanilla

Chocolate No-Butter Buttercream Frosting (page 202)

*Or use any all-purpose gluten-free flour blend that does not contain xanthan gum.

1. Preheat oven to 350°F. Grease and flour two 9-inch round cake pans.

2. Whisk flour blend, sugar, cocoa, baking soda, xanthan gum and salt in large bowl. Combine soymilk, oil, vinegar and vanilla in small bowl.

3. Pour wet ingredients into dry; stir until smooth, scraping bottom and side of bowl. Immediately pour into prepared pans and place in oven.

4. Bake 25 to 30 minutes or until toothpick inserted into centers comes out clean. (Middle of cake may look darker than edges.) Cool in pans on wire rack 5 minutes. Carefully invert onto wire rack; cool completely.

5. Meanwhile, prepare Chocolate No-Butter Buttercream Frosting. Frost cake and decorate as desired.

Makes 10 servings

continued on page 202

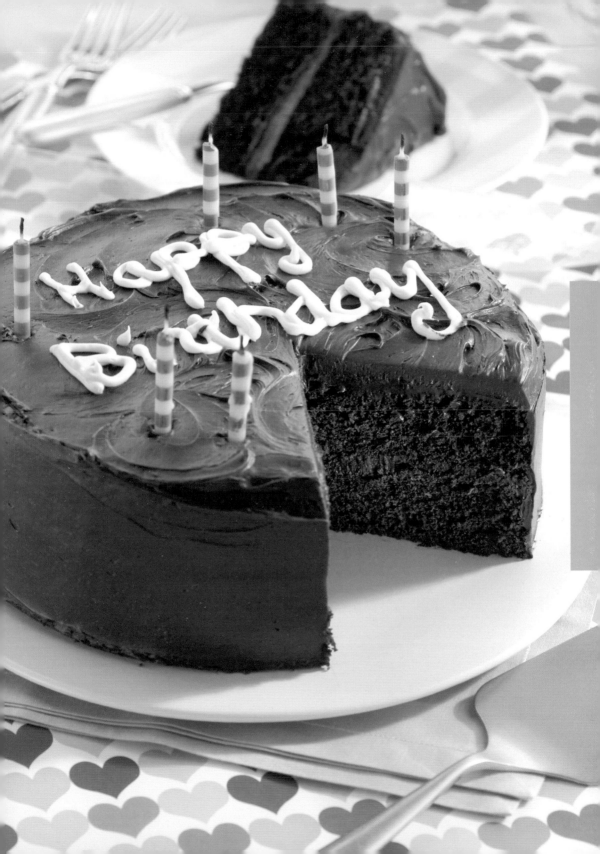

Chocolate No-Butter Buttercream Frosting

¾ cup (1½ sticks) dairy-free margarine
2 teaspoons vanilla
4 cups powdered sugar
½ cup unsweetened cocoa powder
4 to 6 tablespoons soy creamer

1. Beat margarine in medium bowl with electric mixer at medium speed until light and fluffy. Beat in vanilla.

2. Gradually beat in powdered sugar and cocoa. Beat in soy creamer by tablespoonfuls until spreadable.

Tip

To turn Chocolate No-Butter Buttercream into Vanilla, simply omit the cocoa powder and add additional powdered sugar as needed to make the frosting spreadable. Of course, if you can tolerate dairy, you can use butter and regular half-and-half instead of the margarine and soy creamer in this recipe.

Breads
Contents

Gluten-Free Baking

Gluten-free baking isn't harder, it's just different. The good/bad news is that you'll probably be doing more baking now that you're gluten-free. That's good because you won't be eating all the high-fructose corn syrup and other questionable ingredients in most packaged breads and cookies. The bad news is that you'll have to find the time. There is a bit of a learning curve to gluten-free baking, so don't be discouraged by a failure. Remember, you probably failed at traditional baking a few times, too! Many products that may not look as beautiful as you would like will still taste very good. You can also turn a total failure into gluten-free crumbs to be used another time.

Think Different

Many batters and doughs look drastically different from their gluten-containing counterparts. They tend to be wetter and stickier. Bread dough is more like a thick, stretchy batter. You can celebrate the fact that you'll never need to knead GF bread dough. That's a good thing, since it's so sticky you'd never be able to! You will need to learn to shape sticky dough by using damp hands or a well-oiled spoon or spatula. Parchment paper can be a real help for lining pans and transporting soft doughs.

You will be using xanthan gum to provide elasticity and hold doughs together. It's important to measure it very carefully. Too much and your baked goods will shrink after baking. You may find a dense, gummy layer of dough near the bottom of the pan.

Smarty Pans

Pans are a critical part of the recipe. Black or dark metal pans can be a problem because they absorb heat more quickly. The recipes in this book were tested in pans and on baking sheets with light, shiny surfaces. If you must use dark pans, try lining them with foil, watch carefully and lower oven temperatures or cooking times if necessary. Disposable aluminum pans work surprisingly well for many recipes.

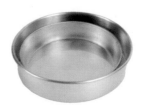

Pan size can be the difference between a perfect cake or loaf and a flop—literally! The same batter intended for a 9×5-inch loaf pan can puff up over the top of an 8×4-inch pan and then collapse. Measure pan size across the top from inside edge to inside edge.

Temperamental Temperatures

Oven temperatures are also important. If you don't have an oven thermometer, you may want to get one. Home ovens are frequently off by as much as 50 degrees. While you're at it, pick up an inexpensive instant-read thermometer, too. It's a big help in knowing when bread is done (190° to 200°F). Gluten-free goods tend to brown more quickly. They can look done on the outside when they're still gooey in the centers so be ready to cover things with a sheet of foil to prevent burning.

Trouble-Shooting

Problem: The cake looked gorgeous when it came out of the oven, but it fell in the center and got mushy.

Solution: Gluten-free baked goods need to be removed from pans quickly or the residual steam can cause them to collapse. Remove them from the pan to a wire rack 5 minutes after they come out of the oven.

Problem: The muffins collapsed over the top of the pan.

Solution: There may have been too much liquid in the batter. Gluten-free flours absorb less liquid than wheat flour.

Problem: The cookies crumbled!

Solution: Did you remember the xanthan gum? Without it GF flours lack the elasticity to hold regular baked goods together.

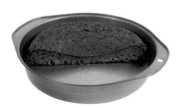

Cake left in a hot pan too long can collapse.

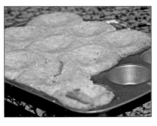

Too much liquid can make muffins collapse.

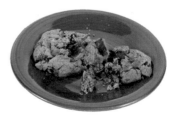

Without xanthan gum, baked goods crumble.

Flour Blends and Friends

Why can't there be a single one-for-one substitute for wheat flour? Unfortunately wheat flour performs many different functions and is made up of both protein (the gluten) and starches. It helps make pie crust flaky, cookies chewy and breads crusty. There is no one GF flour that can recreate all those benefits, but that's no reason to give up baking. With two basic flour blends in your refrigerator you can turn out yummy cakes, cookies and even yeast breads. Here are the blends used for many of the recipes in this book.

Gluten-Free All-Purpose Flour Blend

1 cup white rice flour
1 cup sorghum flour
1 cup tapioca flour
1 cup cornstarch
1 cup almond flour or coconut flour

Combine all ingredients in large bowl. Whisk to make sure flours are evenly distributed. The recipe can be doubled or tripled. Store in airtight container in the refrigerator. *Makes about 5 cups*

Gluten-Free Flour Blend for Breads

1 cup brown rice flour
1 cup sorghum flour
1 cup tapioca flour
1 cup cornstarch
¾ cup millet flour*
⅓ cup instant mashed potato flakes
*If millet flour is not available substitute chickpea flour.

Combine all ingredients in large bowl. Whisk to make sure ingredients are evenly distributed. The recipe can be doubled or tripled. Store in airtight container in the refrigerator. *Makes about 5 cups*

What Is Xanthan Gum Anyway?

It sounds mysterious, doesn't it? Xanthan gum is a chain of polysaccharides (for the nonchemists that's a chain of sugars) made by fermenting a carbohydrate (often corn sugar). Xanthan gum was approved for use as a food additive in 1968 and is used as a thickener and stabilizer in salad dressings, ice cream, low-fat dairy products and, of course, gluten-free baked goods.

If you use a store-bought flour blend, be sure to check the ingredients. Some contain xanthan or guar gum already. You do not want to double the amount of gum in a recipe. The recipes in this book assume that you are using a blend WITHOUT xanthan or guar gum.

Blending the Rules

While gluten-free flour blends may seem mysterious at first, they do follow certain rules. Basic all-purpose flour blends usually start with 2 parts of grain flour (rice, sorghum or millet), 2 parts of starch (cornstarch or tapioca flour) and 1 part of protein (a bean or nut flour). There are many other considerations. Flavor is one. Nutrition is also important. While a blend made of white rice flour and cornstarch might work, it wouldn't contain much in the way of fiber, protein or vitamins. You can, of course, purchase ready-made blends at the supermarket or on the Internet, but homemade is certainly cheaper and also fresher and better tasting.

Storing and Using GF Flour Blends

Most gluten-free flour blends should be stored in the refrigerator or freezer since they contain perishable whole grain or nut flours. Invest in canisters or use clearly marked resealable freezer bags. Bring flours to room temperature before using and remember to rewhisk or shake them so that they are completely combined.

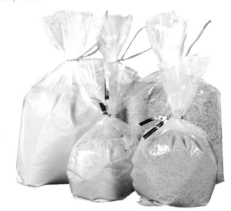

Measuring GF blends is no different than measuring wheat flour, but it is even more important to be accurate. Never pack flour into a measuring cup. Don't dip the measuring cup into the flour, either, since that can compact it. Fluff the flour and spoon it into the cup. Level off the top with the back of a knife.

the Daily Loaf

Sandwich Bread

**3 cups Gluten-Free Flour Blend for Breads (page 206), plus additional
  for pan**
2 packages (¼ ounce each) active dry yeast
2 teaspoons xanthan gum
1 teaspoon salt
1 cup warm water, plus additional as needed
¼ cup vegetable oil
2 eggs
1 tablespoon honey
1 teaspoon cider vinegar

1. Line 9×5-inch loaf pan with foil, dull side out. (Do not use glass loaf pan.)
Extend sides of foil 3 inches up from top of pan. Spray with nonstick cooking
spray and sprinkle with flour blend.

2. Combine 3 cups flour blend, yeast, xanthan gum and salt in large bowl.
Whisk 1 cup water, oil, eggs, honey and vinegar in medium bowl. Beat into
dry ingredients with electric mixer at low speed until batter is smooth, shiny
and thick. Add more water by tablespoonfuls if needed. Beat at medium-high
speed 5 minutes, scraping bowl occasionally.

3. Spoon batter into prepared pan. Cover with lightly oiled plastic wrap; let rise
in warm place 30 minutes or until batter reaches top of pan.

4. Preheat oven to 375°F. Bake 30 to 35 minutes or until bread sounds hollow
when tapped and internal temperature is 200°F. Remove from pan and cool on
wire rack. *Makes 1 (9-inch) loaf*

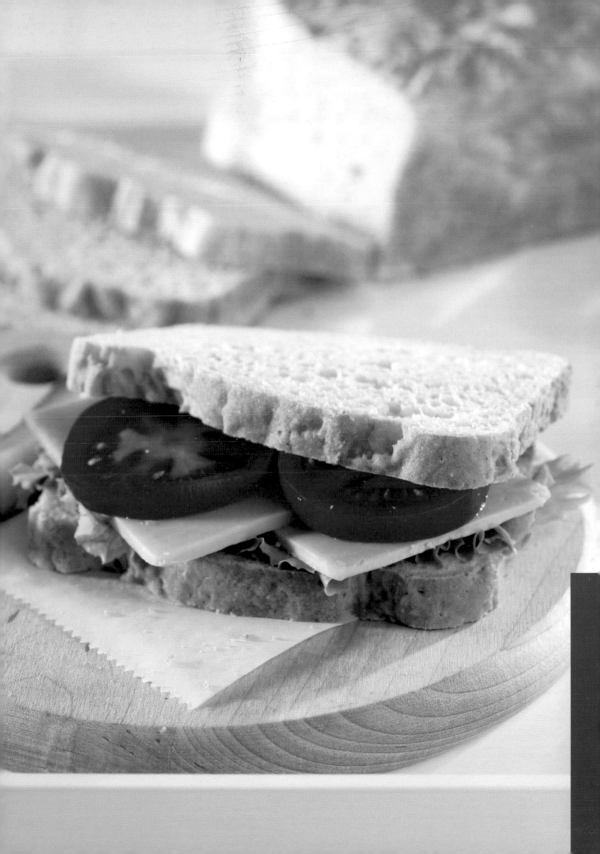

Arepas (Latin American Corn Cakes)

1½ cups instant corn flour for arepas*
½ teaspoon salt
1½ to 2 cups hot water
⅓ cup shredded Mexican cheese blend
1 tablespoon butter, melted
Fillings: scrambled eggs, cheese and salsa

*This corn flour is also called masarepa, masa al instante and harina precodica. It is NOT the same as masa harina or regular cornmeal. Purchase arepa flour at Latin American markets or on the Internet.

1. Preheat oven to 350°F. Mix flour and salt in medium bowl. Stir in 1½ cups hot water. Dough should be smooth and moist but not sticky. Add more water by tablespoonfuls if needed. Add cheese and butter. Knead until dough is consistency of smooth mashed potatoes.

2. Preheat heavy skillet or griddle over medium heat. Grease lightly with butter or oil. Break off a piece of dough about the size of an egg; roll dough into a ball. (If dough cracks or seems too dry, return to bowl and add additional water by tablespoonfuls.) Flatten and pat into 3- to 4-inch disc about ½ inch thick. Immediately place in hot skillet. Repeat with remaining dough.

3. Cook arepas 3 to 5 minutes per side until browned in spots. Transfer to baking sheet. Bake 15 minutes or until arepas sound hollow when tapped.

4. To make breakfast sandwiches, split arepas by piercing edges with fork as you would English muffins. Fill with eggs, cheese and salsa as desired.

Makes 6 to 8 arepas

Note: Arepas are best served warm. Day-old arepas are best toasted. Arepas may also be frozen for future use.

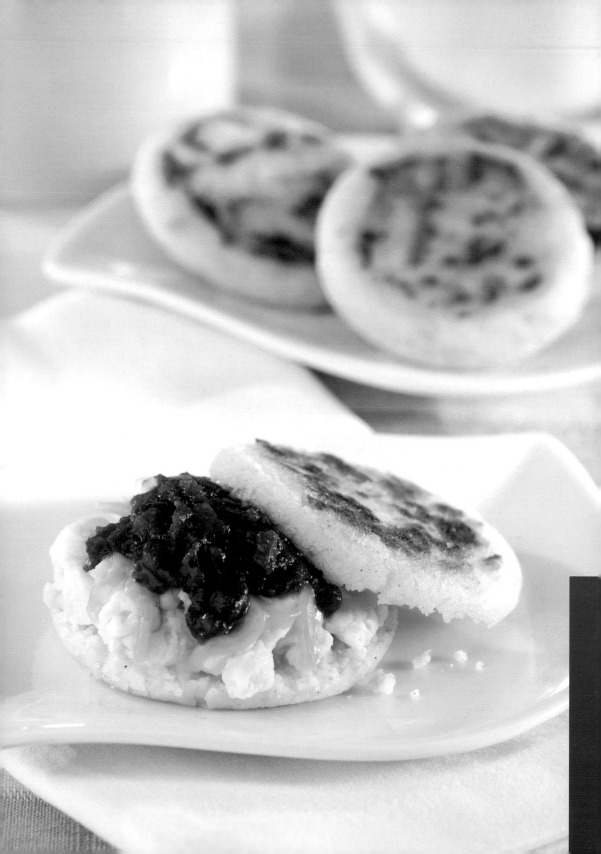

Cinnamon Raisin Bread

3 cups Gluten-Free Flour Blend for Breads (page 206), plus additional
    for pan

2 packages (¼ ounce each) active dry yeast

2 teaspoons xanthan gum

1 teaspoon salt

1¼ cups plus 2 tablespoons warm milk, divided

¼ cup vegetable oil

2 eggs

1 tablespoon honey or maple syrup

1 teaspoon cider vinegar

¾ cup raisins

⅓ cup sugar

1 tablespoon ground cinnamon

1 tablespoon gluten-free oats (optional)

1. Line 9×5-inch loaf pan with foil, dull side out. (Do not use glass loaf pan.) Extend sides of foil 3 inches up from top of pan. Spray with nonstick cooking spray and sprinkle with flour blend.

2. Combine 3 cups flour blend, yeast, xanthan gum and salt in large bowl. Whisk 1¼ cups milk, oil, eggs, honey and vinegar in medium bowl. Beat milk mixture into dry ingredients with electric mixer at low speed until batter is smooth, shiny and thick. Beat at medium-high speed 5 minutes, scraping bowl occasionally. Stir in raisins.

3. Place large sheet of parchment paper on counter; sprinkle with flour blend. Scoop batter onto center of paper. Spread batter with dampened hands or back of oiled spatula to 9×18-inch rectangle. Brush remaining 2 tablespoons milk over dough. Combine sugar and cinnamon in small bowl. Sprinkle all but 1 tablespoon mixture over dough, leaving 1-inch border; lightly press into dough.

4. Using parchment, roll dough jelly-roll style beginning at short end. Push ends in to fit length of pan and trim excess parchment paper. Lift roll using parchment and place in prepared pan. (Leave parchment in pan.) Sprinkle with remaining cinnamon-sugar and oats, if desired.

continued on page 214

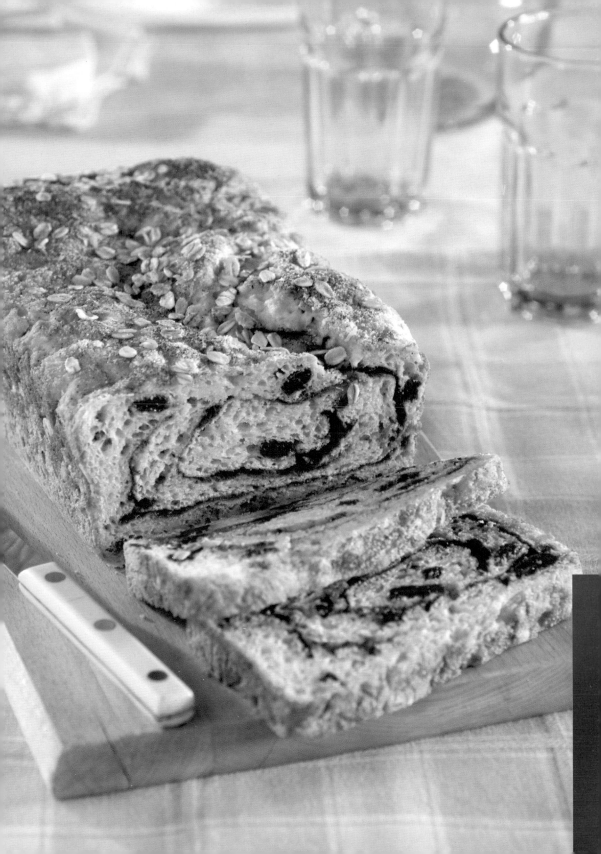

5. Cover loaf with lightly oiled plastic wrap; let rise in warm place 20 to 30 minutes or until batter reaches top of pan.

6. Preheat oven to 375°F. Bake 35 to 45 minutes or until bread sounds hollow when tapped and internal temperature is 200°F. Remove from pan; remove parchment and foil. Cool on wire rack. *Makes 1 (9-inch) loaf*

Brazilian Cheese Rolls (Pão de Queijo)

1 cup whole milk
¼ cup (½ stick) butter, cut into pieces
¼ cup vegetable oil
2 cups plus 2 tablespoons tapioca flour
2 eggs
1 cup grated Parmesan cheese or other firm cheese

1. Preheat oven to 350°F.

2. Combine milk, butter and oil in large saucepan. Bring to a boil over medium heat, stirring to melt butter. Once mixture reaches a boil, remove from heat. Stir in tapioca flour. Mixture will be thick and stretchy.

3. Stir in eggs, one at a time, and cheese. Mixture will be very stiff. Cool mixture in pan until easy to handle.

4. Take heaping tablespoons of dough with tapioca-floured hands and roll into 1½-inch balls. Place on baking sheet about 1 inch apart.

5. Bake 20 to 25 minutes or until puffed and golden. Serve warm.

Makes about 20 rolls

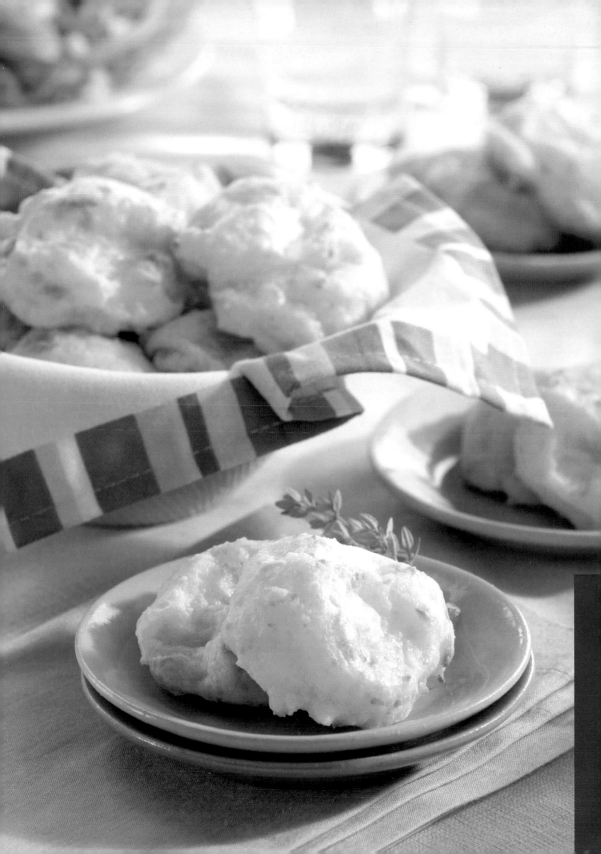

Rosemary Bread

2½ cups Gluten-Free Flour Blend for Breads (page 206), plus additional for pan

  1 tablespoon active dry yeast (about 1½ packages)

  1 tablespoon chopped fresh rosemary leaves

1½ teaspoons xanthan gum

  1 teaspoon unflavored gelatin

 ½ teaspoon salt

  2 eggs

 ¼ cup extra virgin olive oil

 ¾ cup warm milk (110°F)*

*Milk should be warm, but not over 120°F, which could kill yeast. Test temperature on inner wrist. Milk should feel warmer than body temperature, not burning hot.

1. Have all ingredients at room temperature. Spray 8×4-inch loaf pan with nonstick cooking spray and sprinkle with flour blend.

2. Combine 2½ cups flour blend, yeast, rosemary, xanthan gum, gelatin and salt in large bowl. Beat eggs and olive oil in small bowl.

3. Beat egg mixture and milk into flour mixture with electric mixer at low speed until combined. Beat at high speed 3 to 4 minutes. Batter should be smooth and stretchy.

4. Spoon batter into prepared pan. Level top with dampened fingers or oiled spoon. Cover loosely; let rise in warm place about 45 minutes or until batter comes within 1 inch of top of pan.

5. Preheat oven to 400°F. Bake 10 minutes. *Reduce oven temperature to 350°F.* Cover bread loosely with foil. Bake 35 to 45 minutes or until bread sounds hollow when tapped and internal temperature is 190°F.

6. Remove bread from pan to wire rack; cool completely. Tightly wrap leftover bread and refrigerate up to 2 days. Freeze for longer storage.

Makes 1 (8-inch) loaf

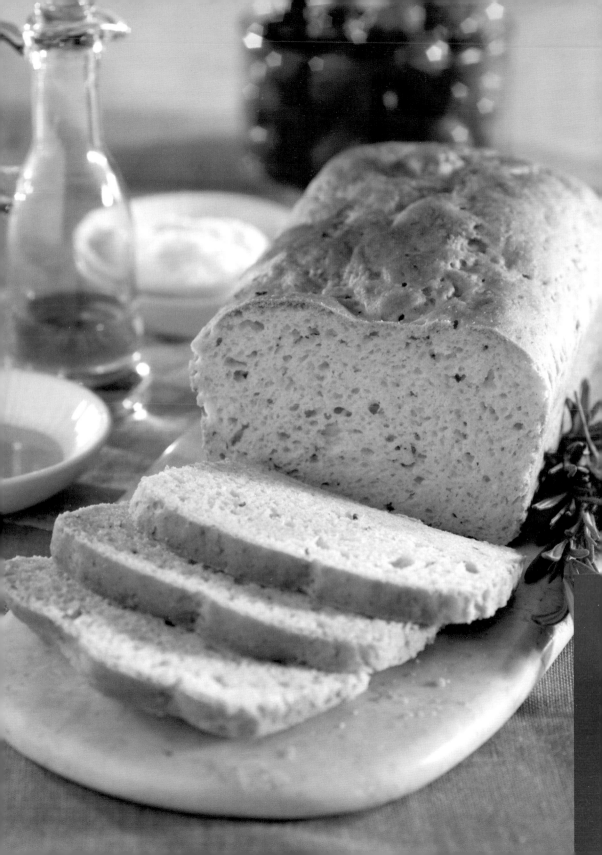

Asiago Garlic Rolls

1 cup warm water (110°F)

1 package (¼ ounce) active dry yeast

1 teaspoon sugar

3 eggs

¼ cup extra virgin olive oil

½ teaspoon cider vinegar

1½ cups Gluten-Free Flour Blend for Breads (page 206)

½ cup cornstarch

¼ cup almond flour

1¼ teaspoons xanthan gum

1 teaspoon unflavored gelatin

½ teaspoon salt

¼ cup plus 2 tablespoons grated Asiago cheese, divided

4 cloves roasted garlic, minced

1 tablespoon chopped fresh rosemary leaves

1. Grease 12 standard (2½-inch) muffin cups. Combine water, yeast and sugar in 2-cup measure; let stand 10 minutes or until foamy. Whisk eggs, olive oil and vinegar in medium bowl.

2. Combine flour blend, cornstarch, almond flour, xanthan gum, gelatin and salt in large bowl. Beat in yeast mixture and egg mixture with electric mixer at low speed. Stir in ¼ cup cheese, garlic and rosemary. Beat at high speed 3 minutes or until smooth.

3. Spoon dough into prepared muffin cups, filling three-fourths full. Cover with plastic wrap sprayed with nonstick cooking spray; let rise in warm place 30 minutes.

4. Preheat oven to 375°F. Sprinkle remaining 2 tablespoons cheese on rolls. Bake 20 to 25 minutes or until lightly browned. Remove rolls from pan and cool on wire rack.   *Makes 12 rolls*

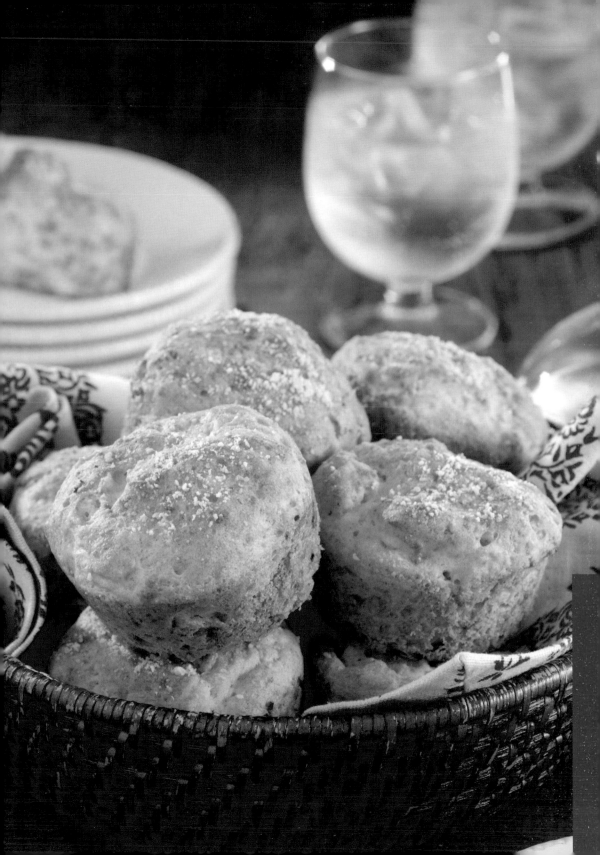

Chili Cheese Bread

¾ **cup water**

2 **eggs**

3 **tablespoons olive oil**

1½ **cups Gluten-Free Flour Blend for Breads (page 206)**

1 **cup (4 ounces) shredded Cheddar cheese**

1 **tablespoon sugar**

1 **tablespoon chili powder**

1 **package (¼ ounce) active dry yeast**

1½ **teaspoons xanthan gum**

1 **teaspoon unflavored gelatin**

½ **teaspoon salt**

1. Grease 8×4-inch loaf pan or spray with nonstick cooking spray.

2. Beat water, eggs and olive oil in large bowl with electric mixer at medium speed until combined. Whisk flour blend, cheese, sugar, chili powder, yeast, xanthan gum, gelatin and salt in large bowl until thoroughly mixed.

3. Gradually beat flour mixture into wet ingredients; beat at low speed 10 minutes. Batter will be sticky and stretchy. Spoon batter into prepared pan.

4. Cover; let rise in warm place about 1 hour or until dough almost reaches top of pan.

5. Preheat oven to 350°F. Bake 40 to 50 minutes or until bread sounds hollow when tapped and internal temperature is 190°F. Check after 20 minutes and cover with foil if bread is browning too quickly. Cool in pan on wire rack 5 minutes. Remove from pan; cool completely before slicing.

Makes 1 (8-inch) loaf

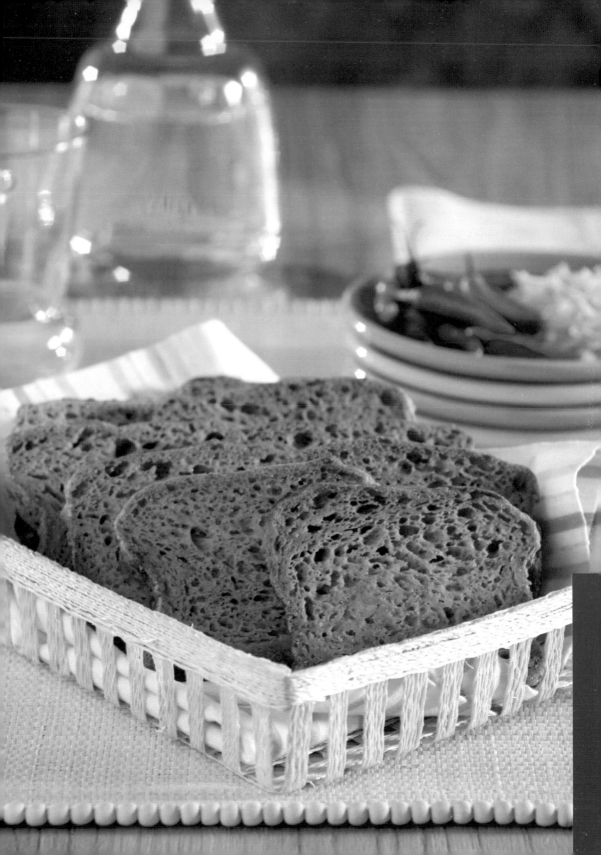

GF Breadsticks

3½ cups Gluten-Free Flour Blend for Breads (page 206)
1 package (¼ ounce) active dry yeast
3 teaspoons salt, divided
1½ teaspoons xanthan gum
1 teaspoon unflavored gelatin
1⅓ cups warm water, plus additional for brushing
2 tablespoons olive oil
1 tablespoon honey
Sesame seeds and/or poppy seeds

Garlic Topping
2 tablespoons olive oil
2 to 4 cloves garlic, minced

1. Place flour blend, yeast, 2 teaspoons salt, xanthan gum and gelatin in food processor; process until mixed.

2. With processor running, add 1⅓ cups water, 2 tablespoons olive oil and honey. Process 30 seconds or until thoroughly combined; dough will be sticky. Transfer to large greased bowl. Shape into rough ball with damp hands. Cover; let rise in warm place 45 minutes. Punch down dough; let rest 15 minutes.

3. Preheat oven to 450°F. Line two large baking sheets with parchment paper. Place 1½-inch balls of dough on clean surface; roll into 8-inch-long breadsticks. Transfer to prepared baking sheet.

4. Brush breadsticks lightly with additional water and sprinkle with seeds. For garlic topping, combine 2 tablespoons olive oil and garlic in small bowl. Brush on breadsticks after 10 minutes of baking.

5. Bake 20 minutes or until breadsticks are browned, rotating pans once during baking. Remove to wire racks to cool slightly. Serve warm.

Makes 15 to 20 breadsticks

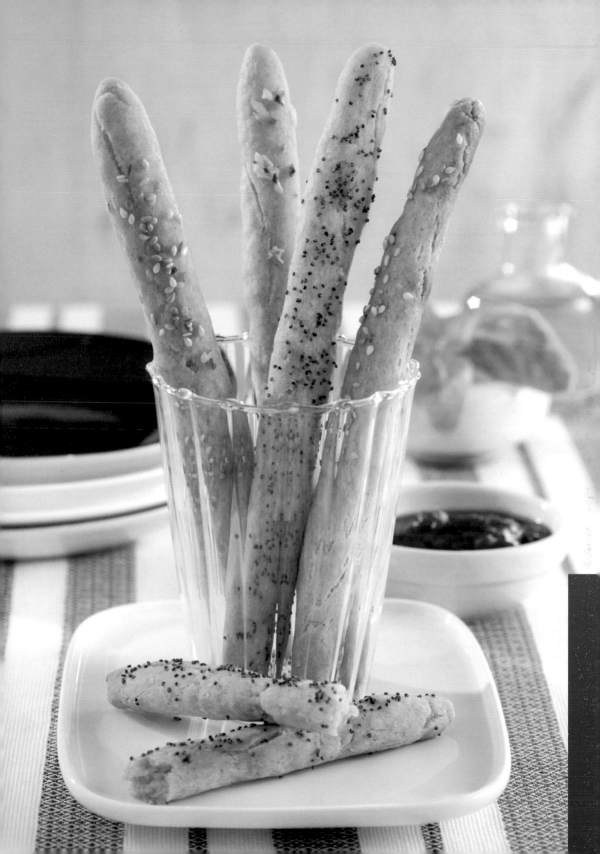

Multigrain Sandwich Bread

1 cup brown rice flour, plus additional for pan
1 tablespoon active dry yeast (about 1½ packages)
1¾ cups warm water (110°F)
2 tablespoons honey
¾ cup white rice flour
⅔ cup dry milk powder
½ cup gluten-free oat flour
⅓ cup cornstarch
⅓ cup potato starch
¼ cup teff flour
2 teaspoons xanthan gum
2 teaspoons egg white powder
1½ teaspoons salt
1 teaspoon gelatin
2 eggs
¼ cup canola oil

1. Preheat oven to 350°F. Grease 10×5-inch loaf pan and sprinkle with brown rice flour.

2. Sprinkle yeast over warm water in medium bowl. Add honey. Cover with plastic wrap; let stand 10 minutes or until foamy.

3. Combine 1 cup brown rice flour, white rice flour, dry milk powder, oat flour, cornstarch, potato starch, teff flour, xanthan gum, egg white powder, salt and gelatin in large bowl. Stir until well blended.

4. Beat eggs in small bowl; whisk in oil.

5. Beat yeast mixture and egg mixture into flour mixture with electric mixer until combined. Beat at high speed 5 minutes or until smooth. Spoon into prepared pan.

6. Bake 1 hour or until internal temperature is 200°F. Remove from pan and cool on wire rack. *Makes 1 (10-inch) loaf*

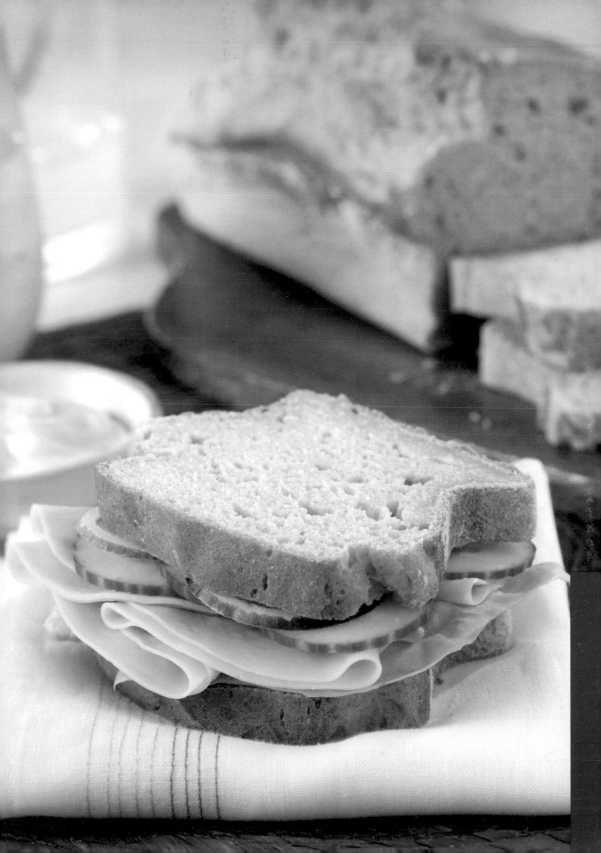

Chili Corn Bread

Nonstick cooking spray
¼ cup chopped red bell pepper
¼ cup chopped green bell pepper
2 small jalapeño peppers,* minced
2 cloves garlic, minced
¾ cup corn
1½ cups yellow cornmeal
½ cup Gluten-Free All-Purpose Flour Blend (page 206)**
2 tablespoons sugar
2 teaspoons baking powder
1½ teaspoons xanthan gum
½ teaspoon baking soda
½ teaspoon salt
½ teaspoon ground cumin
1½ cups buttermilk
1 egg
2 egg whites
¼ cup (½ stick) butter, melted

*Jalapeño peppers can sting and irritate the skin, so wear rubber gloves when handling peppers and do not touch your eyes.

**Or use any all-purpose gluten-free flour blend that does not contain xanthan gum.

1. Preheat oven to 375°F. Spray 8-inch square baking pan with cooking spray.

2. Spray small skillet with cooking spray. Add bell peppers, jalapeños and garlic; cook and stir over medium heat 3 to 4 minutes or until peppers are tender. Stir in corn; cook 1 to 2 minutes. Remove from heat.

3. Combine cornmeal, flour blend, sugar, baking powder, xanthan gum, baking soda, salt and cumin in large bowl. Add buttermilk, egg, egg whites and butter; mix until blended. Stir in corn mixture. Pour batter into prepared pan.

4. Bake 25 to 30 minutes or until golden brown. Cool in pan on wire rack.

Makes 12 servings

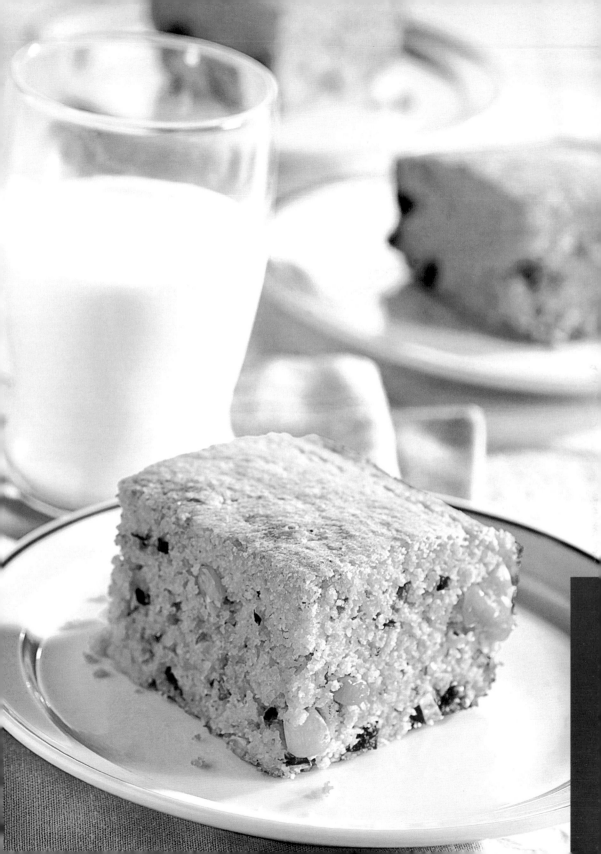

Muffins & More

Gluten-Free Corn Muffins

....

   1 cup Gluten-Free All-Purpose Flour Blend (page 206)*
   1 cup cornmeal
   ½ cup sugar
1½ teaspoons baking powder
   1 teaspoon baking soda
   ½ teaspoon salt
   ½ teaspoon xanthan gum
   1 cup buttermilk
   ¼ cup (½ stick) butter, melted
   2 eggs

Or use any all-purpose gluten-free flour blend that does not contain xanthan gum.

1. Preheat oven to 350°F. Grease 12 standard (2½-inch) muffin cups or line with paper baking cups.

2. Combine flour blend, cornmeal, sugar, baking powder, baking soda, salt and xanthan gum in large bowl. Whisk buttermilk, butter and eggs in medium bowl. Add to dry ingredients and blend well. Batter will be thick.

3. Spoon batter into prepared muffin cups, filling almost to top. Bake muffins 20 to 25 minutes or until lightly browned and toothpick inserted into centers comes out clean. Cool in pan 5 minutes; remove to wire rack. Serve warm.

Makes 12 muffins

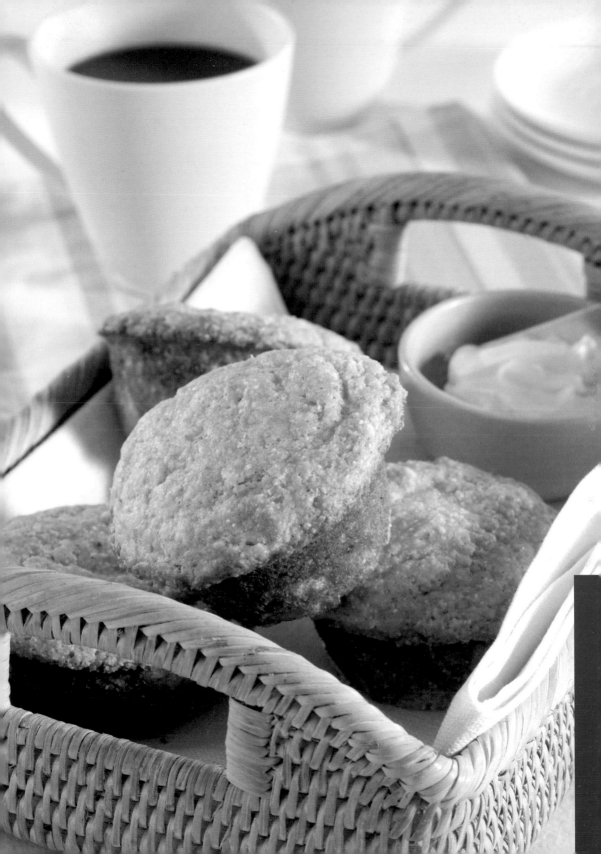

Loaded Banana Bread

6 tablespoons shortening

⅓ cup packed light brown sugar

⅓ cup granulated sugar

1 egg

3 ripe bananas, mashed

½ teaspoon vanilla

1½ cups Gluten-Free All-Purpose Flour Blend (page 206)*

2½ teaspoons baking powder

1 teaspoon xanthan gum

½ teaspoon salt

1 can (8 ounces) crushed pineapple, drained

⅓ cup flaked coconut

⅓ cup semisweet chocolate chips

⅓ cup chopped walnuts

*Or use any all-purpose gluten-free flour blend that does not contain xanthan gum.

1. Preheat oven to 350°F. Coat 9×5-inch loaf pan with nonstick cooking spray.

2. Beat shortening, brown sugar and granulated sugar in large bowl with electric mixer at medium speed until light and fluffy. Beat in egg, bananas and vanilla just until combined.

3. Stir flour blend, baking powder, xanthan gum and salt in small bowl. Gradually beat flour mixture into banana mixture just until combined. Stir in pineapple, coconut and chocolate chips.

4. Spoon batter into prepared pan. Top with walnuts. Bake 50 to 60 minutes or until toothpick inserted into center comes out almost clean. Cool in pan 5 minutes; transfer to wire rack.

Makes 1 (9-inch) loaf

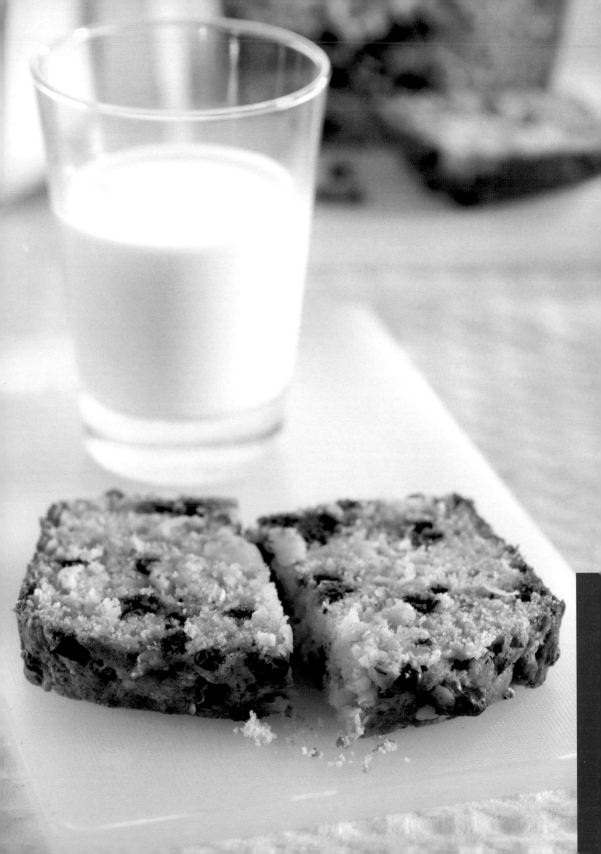

Snacking Surprise Muffins

⅔ cup rice milk or other milk

2 teaspoons cider vinegar

1½ cups Gluten-Free All-Purpose Flour Blend (page 206)*

1 cup fresh or frozen blueberries

½ cup plus 1 tablespoon sugar, divided

1 tablespoon baking powder

1¼ teaspoons ground cinnamon, divided

½ teaspoon xanthan gum

¼ teaspoon salt

1 egg, beaten

¼ cup (½ stick) dairy-free margarine, melted

3 tablespoons peach or apricot preserves

Or use any all-purpose gluten-free flour blend that does not contain xanthan gum.

1. Preheat oven to 400°F. Line 12 standard (2½-inch) muffin cups with paper baking cups.

2. Combine rice milk and vinegar in small bowl; let stand 10 minutes. Meanwhile, combine flour blend, blueberries, ½ cup sugar, baking powder, 1 teaspoon cinnamon, xanthan gum and salt in medium bowl. Add rice milk mixture, egg and margarine to flour mixture; mix just until moistened.

3. Spoon about 1 tablespoon batter into each prepared muffin cup. Drop a scant teaspoonful of preserves into center of batter in each cup; top with remaining batter.

4. Combine remaining 1 tablespoon sugar and ¼ teaspoon cinnamon in small bowl; sprinkle evenly over batter.

5. Bake 18 to 20 minutes or until lightly browned. Remove muffins to wire rack to cool completely.   *Makes 12 muffins*

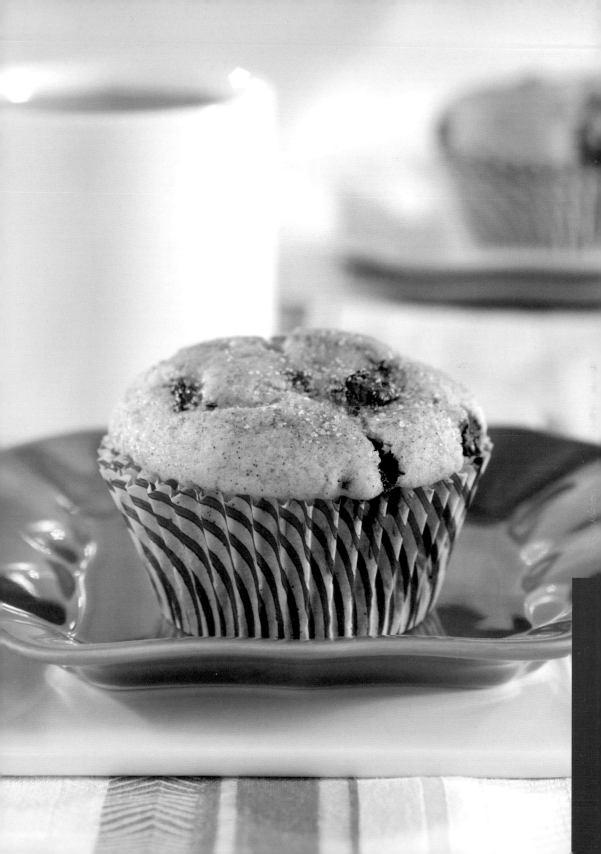

Applesauce Muffins

2 cups Gluten-Free All-Purpose Flour Blend (page 206)*
½ cup plus 3 tablespoons granulated sugar, divided
½ cup plus 3 tablespoons packed brown sugar, divided
4 teaspoons ground cinnamon, divided
2 teaspoons baking powder
1 teaspoon baking soda
1 teaspoon xanthan gum
½ cup chunky applesauce
½ cup vegetable oil
½ cup apple cider
2 eggs
3 tablespoons dairy-free margarine
Powdered sugar

*Or use any all-purpose gluten-free flour blend that does not contain xanthan gum.

1. Preheat oven to 350°F. Line 16 standard (2½-inch) muffin cups with paper baking cups.

2. Combine flour blend, ½ cup granulated sugar, ½ cup brown sugar, 3 teaspoons cinnamon, baking powder, baking soda and xanthan gum in large bowl. Add applesauce, oil, apple cider and eggs; mix well.

3. For topping, stir remaining 3 tablespoons granulated sugar, 3 tablespoons brown sugar, 1 teaspoon cinnamon and margarine in small bowl with fork until small clumps form.

4. Fill prepared muffin cups two-thirds full with batter. Sprinkle with topping. Bake on center rack 25 to 30 minutes. Cool in pans on wire racks 5 minutes; remove from pans to cool completely. Dust tops with powdered sugar.

Makes 16 muffins

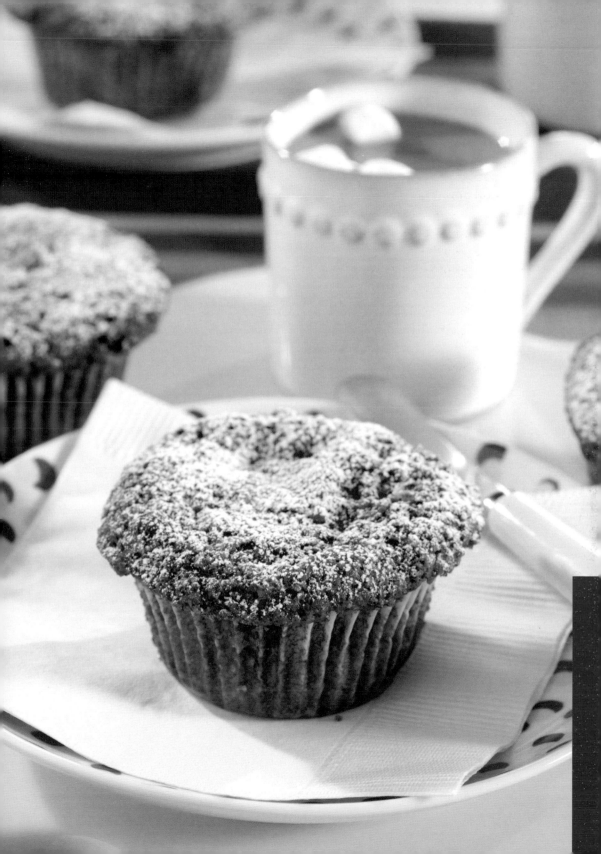

Piña Colada Muffins

....

2 cups **Gluten-Free All-Purpose Flour Blend (page 206)***

¾ **cup sugar**

½ **cup flaked coconut**

1 **tablespoon baking powder**

1 **teaspoon xanthan gum**

½ **teaspoon baking soda**

½ **teaspoon salt**

2 **eggs**

1 **cup sour cream**

1 **can (8 ounces) crushed pineapple in juice, undrained**

¼ **cup (½ stick) butter, melted**

⅛ **teaspoon coconut extract**

Additional flaked coconut (optional)

Or use any all-purpose gluten-free flour blend that does not contain xanthan gum.

1. Preheat oven to 400°F. Spray 18 standard (2½-inch) muffin cups with nonstick cooking spray or line with paper baking cups.

2. Combine flour blend, sugar, coconut, baking powder, xanthan gum, baking soda and salt in large bowl; mix well.

3. Beat eggs in medium bowl with electric mixer at medium speed 1 to 2 minutes or until frothy. Beat in sour cream, pineapple with juice, butter and coconut extract. Stir into flour mixture just until combined. Spoon batter into prepared muffin cups, filling three-fourths full.

4. Bake 15 to 20 minutes or until toothpick inserted into centers comes out clean. If desired, sprinkle tops of muffins with additional coconut after first 10 minutes. Cool in pans 2 minutes. Remove to wire racks; cool completely.

Makes 18 muffins

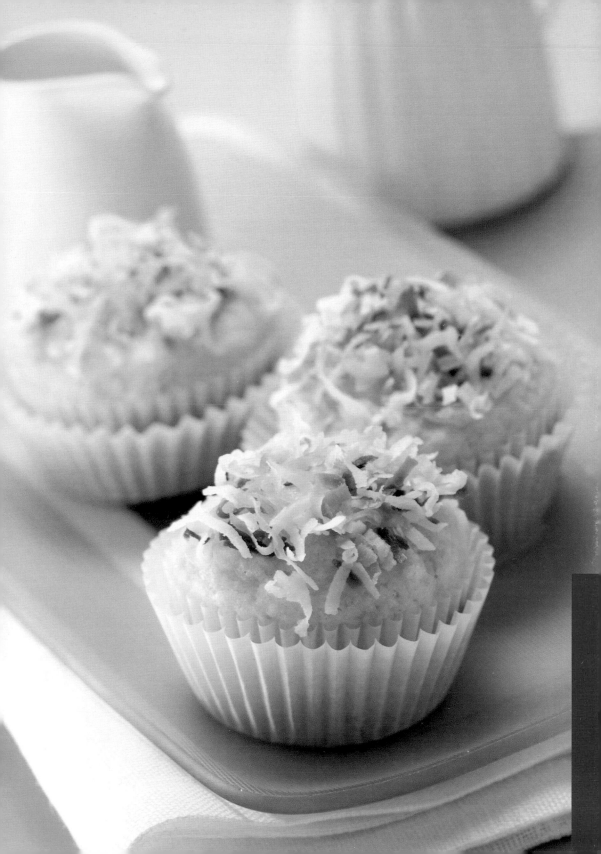

Corn and Sunflower Seed Biscuits

2 cups gluten-free biscuit baking mix
1 tablespoon sugar
2 teaspoons baking powder
½ teaspoon salt
½ teaspoon dried thyme
5 tablespoons dairy-free margarine
1 cup rice milk or other milk
1 cup corn*
⅓ cup plus 5 teaspoons salted roasted sunflower seeds, divided

*Use fresh or thawed frozen corn; do not use supersweet corn.

1. Preheat oven to 400°F. Line baking sheet with parchment paper or coat with nonstick cooking spray.

2. Combine baking mix, sugar, baking powder, salt and thyme in large bowl. Cut in margarine with pastry blender or two knives until mixture resembles coarse crumbs. Add rice milk; stir gently to form soft sticky dough. Stir in corn and ⅓ cup sunflower seeds. Drop dough by ¼ cupfuls onto prepared baking sheet. Sprinkle ½ teaspoon sunflower seeds on each biscuit.

3. Bake 18 to 20 minutes or until golden. Transfer to wire rack to cool slightly. Serve warm.

Makes 12 biscuits

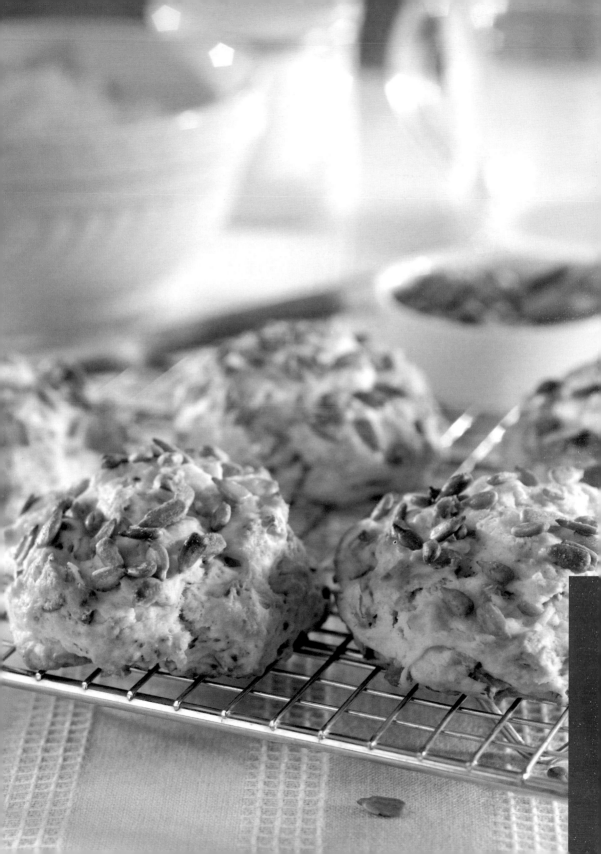

Blueberry Coconut Flour Muffins

6 eggs
½ cup sugar
¼ cup (½ stick) butter, melted
¼ cup milk
½ cup plus 2 teaspoons coconut flour,* divided
2 teaspoons grated lemon peel
½ teaspoon salt
½ teaspoon baking powder
½ teaspoon xanthan gum
1 cup blueberries

*Coconut flour is available in the specialty flour section of many supermarkets. It can also be ordered on the Internet.

1. Preheat oven to 375°F. Grease 12 standard (2½-inch) muffin cups or line with paper liners.

2. Whisk eggs, sugar, butter and milk in medium bowl until well combined.

3. Thoroughly combine ½ cup coconut flour, lemon peel, salt, baking powder and xanthan gum in medium bowl. Sift flour mixture into egg mixture. Whisk until batter is smooth.

4. Combine blueberries with remaining 2 teaspoons coconut flour in small bowl. Stir gently into batter.

5. Fill prepared muffin cups almost full. Bake 12 to 15 minutes or until toothpick inserted into centers comes out clean. Cool in pan on wire rack 5 minutes. Remove from pan and serve warm.   *Makes 12 muffins*

Tip: Coconut flour is a gluten-free, high-fiber, low-carbohydrate flour that adds a touch of sweetness to these muffins. Because it absorbs a great deal of liquid, a little coconut flour goes a long way. Most recipes using it also call for more eggs than usual since it can become heavy without the extra lift that eggs provide.

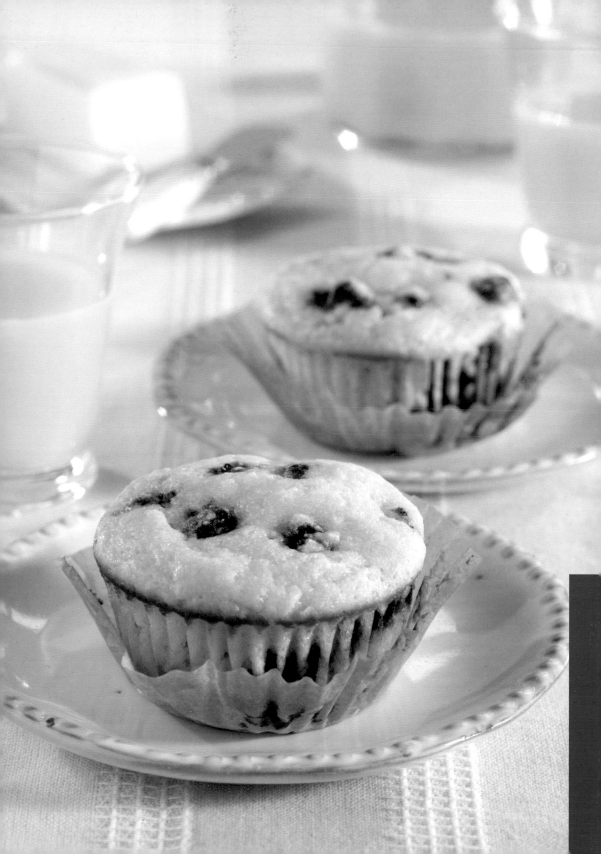

Taco Boulders

2¼ **cups gluten-free biscuit baking mix**
1 **cup (4 ounces) shredded taco cheese blend**
2 **tablespoons diced mild green chiles**
⅔ **cup milk**
3 **tablespoons butter, melted**
¼ **teaspoon chili powder**
¼ **teaspoon garlic powder**

1. Preheat oven to 425°F. Line baking sheet with parchment paper or spray with nonstick cooking spray.

2. Combine baking mix, cheese and chiles in large bowl. Stir in milk just until moistened. Drop dough by ¼ cupfuls into 12 mounds on prepared baking sheet.

3. Bake 11 to 13 minutes or until golden brown. Meanwhile, combine butter, chili powder and garlic powder in small bowl. Remove biscuits to wire rack; immediately brush with butter mixture. Serve warm.   *Makes 12 biscuits*

Tip

When you use premade gluten-free baking products, you may still want to check the ingredients list. There won't be any wheat flour or gluten, but there may be other ingredients you wish to avoid. Blends can be made from a huge variety of flours, including soy, corn, potato, almond, chickpea and many others.

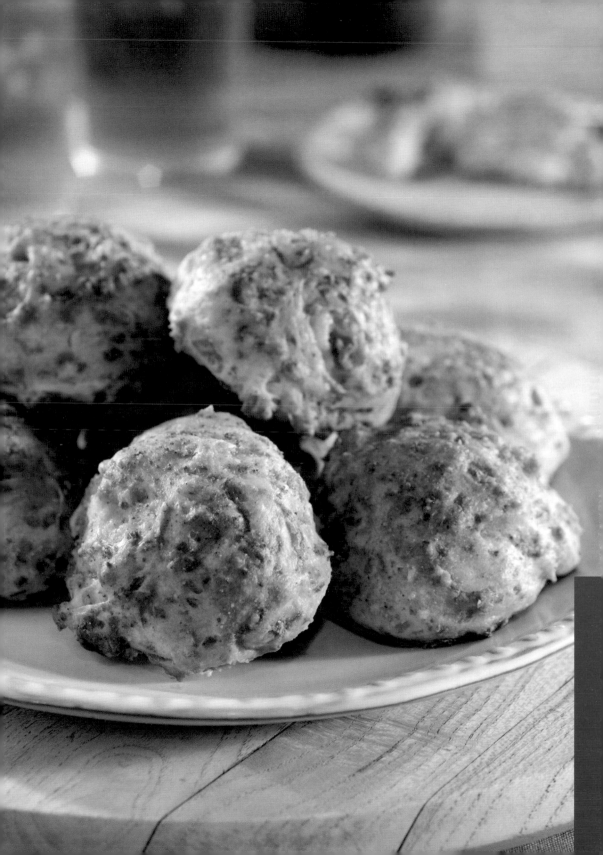

Spiced Sweet Potato Muffins

⅓ cup plus 2 tablespoons packed brown sugar, divided

2 teaspoons ground cinnamon, divided

1½ cups Gluten-Free All-Purpose Flour Blend (page 206)*

1 tablespoon baking powder

½ teaspoon salt

½ teaspoon baking soda

½ teaspoon ground allspice

½ teaspoon xanthan gum

1 cup mashed cooked sweet potatoes

¾ cup rice milk or other milk

¼ cup vegetable oil

¼ cup unsweetened applesauce

Or use any all-purpose gluten-free flour blend that does not contain xanthan gum.

1. Preheat oven to 425°F. Grease 12 standard (2½-inch) muffin cups.

2. Combine 2 tablespoons brown sugar and 1 teaspoon cinnamon in small bowl; set aside.

3. Combine flour blend, baking powder, remaining 1 teaspoon cinnamon, salt, baking soda, allspice and xanthan gum in large bowl. Stir in remaining ⅓ cup brown sugar.

4. Combine sweet potatoes, rice milk, oil and applesauce in medium bowl. Stir into flour mixture just until moistened. Spoon evenly into prepared muffin cups. Sprinkle with cinnamon mixture.

5. Bake 14 to 16 minutes or until toothpick inserted into centers comes out clean. Remove to wire rack; cool completely.   *Makes 12 muffins*

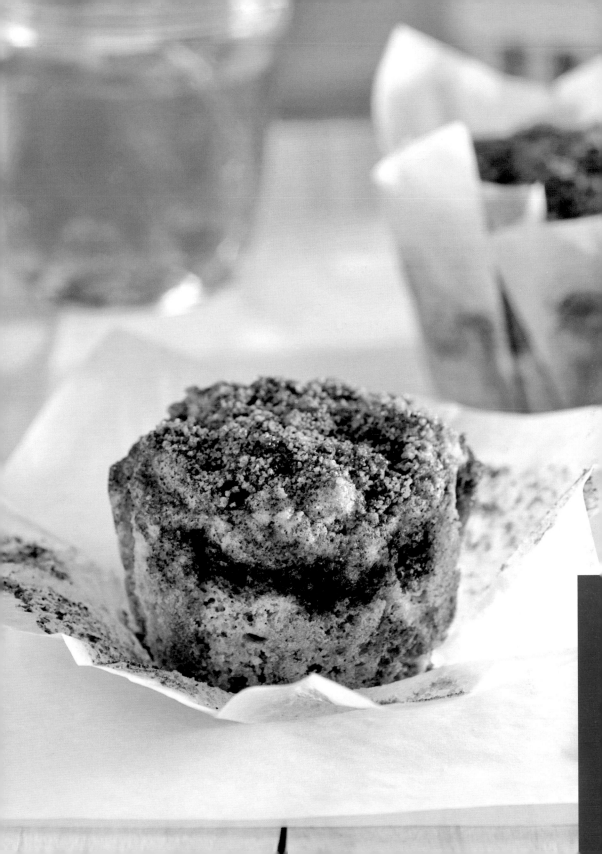

Cinnamon Scones

2 cups Gluten-Free All-Purpose Flour Blend (page 206),* plus additional for work surface

¼ cup sugar

2½ teaspoons baking powder

¾ teaspoon salt

¾ teaspoon xanthan gum

½ teaspoon baking soda

⅓ cup cinnamon chips

½ cup (1 stick) cold butter, cut into small pieces

½ cup plain yogurt

¾ cup milk

2 tablespoons cinnamon-sugar

*Or use any all-purpose gluten-free flour blend that does not contain xanthan gum.

1. Preheat oven to 425°F.

2. Combine flour blend, sugar, baking powder, salt, xanthan gum and baking soda in large bowl. Add cinnamon chips and toss to combine.

3. Cut butter into flour mixture with pastry blender or two knives until coarse crumbs form. Stir yogurt into milk in small bowl or large measuring cup until combined.

4. Gradually add wet ingredients to dry ingredients, stirring just until dough begins to form. (You may not need all of yogurt mixture.) Transfer to surface sprinkled with flour blend. Knead 5 or 6 times until dough holds together. Divide into 2 pieces.

5. Pat each dough piece into 5-inch circle about ½ inch thick. Cut each circle into 6 wedges with floured knife. Place scones 2 inches apart on baking sheets. Sprinkle with cinnamon-sugar.

6. Bake 10 to 14 minutes or until lightly browned. Cool on wire rack.

Makes 12 scones

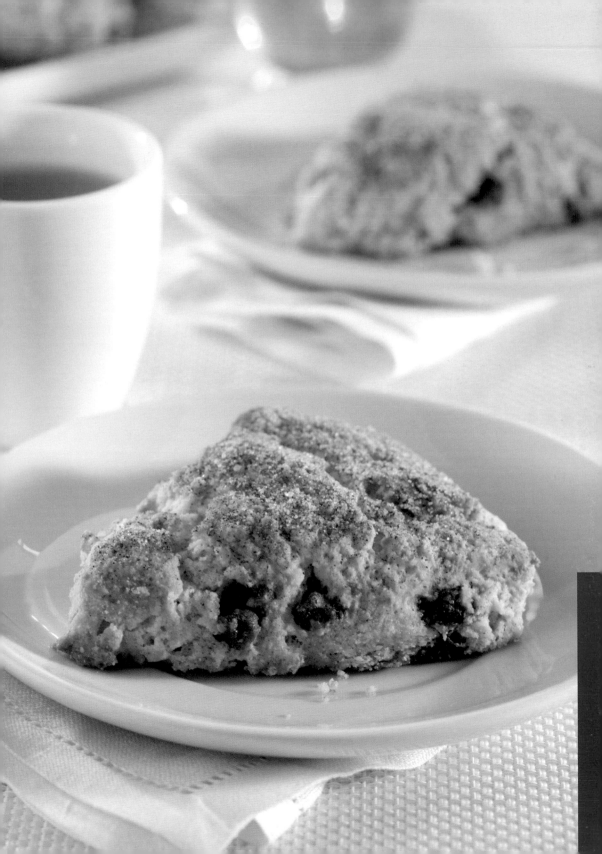

Flavorful Flatbreads

Wild West Pizza

. . . .

3 cups Gluten-Free Flour Blend for Breads (page 206)

2 packages (¼ ounce each) active dry yeast

2 teaspoons xanthan gum

1 teaspoon salt

1 cup warm water

¼ cup extra virgin olive oil

3 egg whites

1 tablespoon honey

1 teaspoon cider vinegar

Toppings

1½ cups gluten-free barbecue sauce

2 cups chopped cooked chicken

½ red onion, cut into thin slivers

1 bell pepper, finely chopped (optional)

1. Preheat oven to 450°F. Line baking sheets or pizza pans with parchment paper.

2. Mix flour blend, yeast, xanthan gum and salt in large bowl. Whisk water, olive oil, egg whites, honey and vinegar in medium bowl. Beat wet ingredients into dry ingredients with electric mixer at low speed until combined. Add additional water by tablespoonfuls until batter is smooth and thick. Beat at medium-high speed 5 minutes, scraping bowl occasionally.

continued on page 250

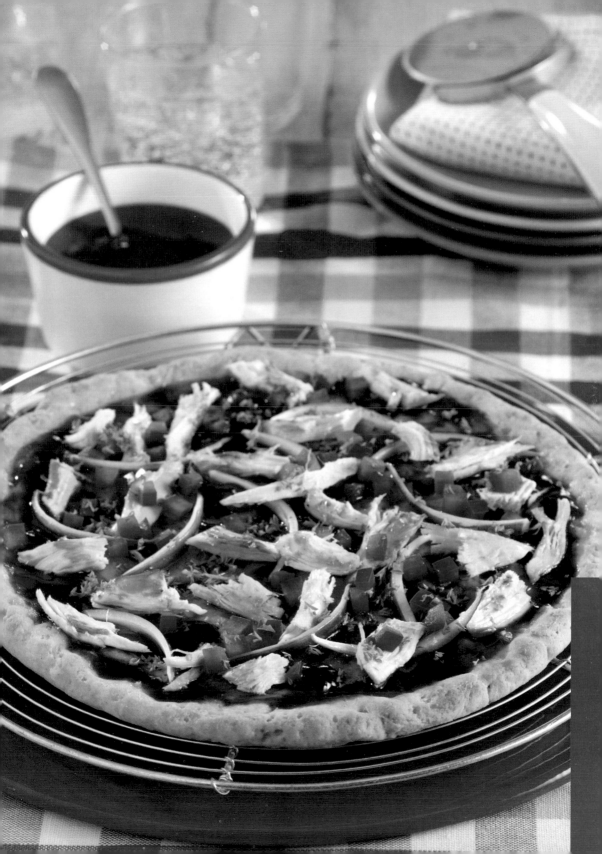

3. Transfer one third of dough to prepared pan. Spread dough into 10-inch circle using dampened fingers or back of oiled spoon, making crust thicker around edge to hold toppings. Repeat with remaining dough.

4. Bake 8 to 10 minutes or until crusts are lightly browned.* Spread crusts with barbecue sauce. Arrange chicken, onion and bell pepper, if desired, on top. Bake 2 to 5 minutes or until heated through. *Makes 3 (10-inch) pizzas*
To freeze pizza crusts for later use, allow them to cool, wrap well and store in the freezer for up to 3 months.

Gluten-Free Waffles

2 **eggs**
½ **cup plain yogurt**
½ **cup milk**
1 **cup Gluten-Free All-Purpose Flour Blend (page 206)***
1 **tablespoon sugar**
1 **teaspoon baking powder**
1 **teaspoon baking soda**
½ **teaspoon salt**
2 **tablespoons butter, melted**
Butter and maple syrup

Or use any all-purpose gluten-free flour blend that does not contain xanthan gum.

1. Preheat waffle iron according to manufacturer's directions.

2. Beat eggs in medium bowl until light and fluffy. Whisk in yogurt and milk.

3. Combine flour blend, sugar, baking powder, baking soda and salt in large bowl. Gradually whisk yogurt mixture into flour mixture until smooth. Whisk in melted butter.

4. Add batter to waffle iron by ½ cupfuls for 6-inch waffles (adjust amount depending on waffle iron). Bake until crisp and browned. Serve with butter and syrup. Refrigerate or freeze leftover waffles; reheat in toaster oven until crisp.
Makes 5 (6-inch) waffles

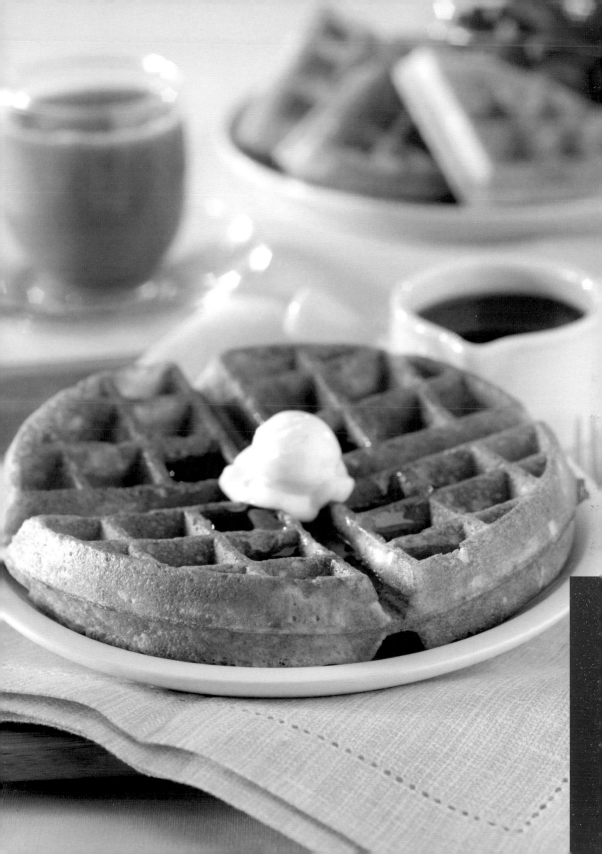

Tomato Zucchini Focaccia

3 cups Gluten-Free Flour Blend for Breads (page 206)

2 packages (¼ ounce each) active dry yeast

1 tablespoon chopped fresh basil

2 teaspoons xanthan gum

1 teaspoon salt

1 cup warm water

¼ cup extra virgin olive oil

3 egg whites

1 tablespoon honey

1 teaspoon cider vinegar

Toppings

2 plum tomatoes, thinly sliced

1 zucchini, thinly sliced

½ cup grated Parmesan cheese

1. Mix flour blend, yeast, basil, xanthan gum and salt in large bowl. Whisk water, olive oil, egg whites, honey and vinegar in medium bowl. Beat wet ingredients into dry ingredients with electric mixer at low speed until combined. Add more water by tablespoonfuls, if needed, until batter is smooth, shiny and thick. Beat at medium-high speed 5 minutes, scraping bowl occasionally.

2. Preheat oven to 450°F. Line baking sheet with parchment paper or foil. Transfer half of dough to prepared baking sheet. Spread into 8-inch round about ½ inch thick using dampened hands. Repeat with remaining dough.

3. Let dough rest 20 minutes. Dimple top of dough with fingertips. Arrange tomatoes and zucchini on each focaccia, pressing in lightly.

4. Bake about 10 minutes or until beginning to brown. Sprinkle with cheese and bake 5 minutes or until cheese melts. *Makes 2 focaccia breads*

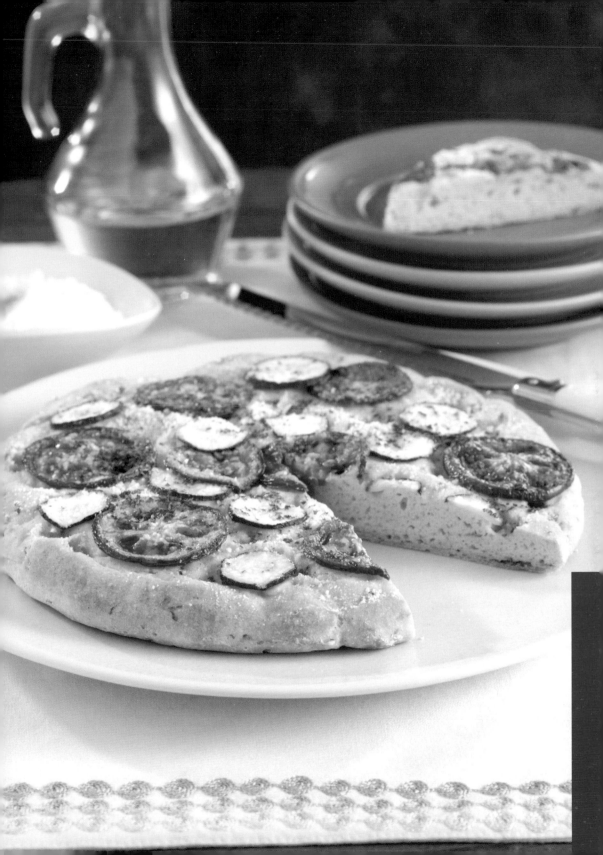

Socca (Niçoise Chickpea Pancake)

1 cup chickpea flour

¾ teaspoon salt

½ teaspoon ground black pepper

1 cup water

5 tablespoons olive oil, divided

1½ teaspoons minced fresh basil *or* ½ teaspoon dried basil

1 teaspoon minced fresh rosemary leaves *or* ¼ teaspoon
    dried rosemary

¼ teaspoon dried thyme

1. Sift chickpea flour into medium bowl. Stir in salt and pepper. Gradually whisk in water to create a smooth batter. Stir in 2 tablespoons olive oil. Allow batter to rest at least 30 minutes.

2. Preheat oven to 450°F about 10 minutes before ready to bake socca. Place 9- or 10-inch cast iron skillet in oven to heat.

3. Add basil, rosemary and thyme to batter; whisk until smooth. Carefully remove skillet from oven using oven mitts. Add 2 tablespoons olive oil to skillet; swirl to coat evenly. Immediately pour in batter.

4. Bake 12 to 15 minutes or until edge begins to pull away and center is firm. Remove skillet; *turn oven to broil.*

5. Brush socca with remaining tablespoon oil and broil 2 to 4 minutes or until dark brown in spots. Cut into wedges and serve warm.   *Makes 6 servings*

Tip: Socca are pancakes made of chickpea flour and are commonly served in paper cones as a savory street food in the south of France, especially around Nice. Chickpea flour can also be used to make crêpes. Increase the amount of water in the recipe by about ¼ cup to make a thinner batter and cook the crêpes in a small nonstick skillet.

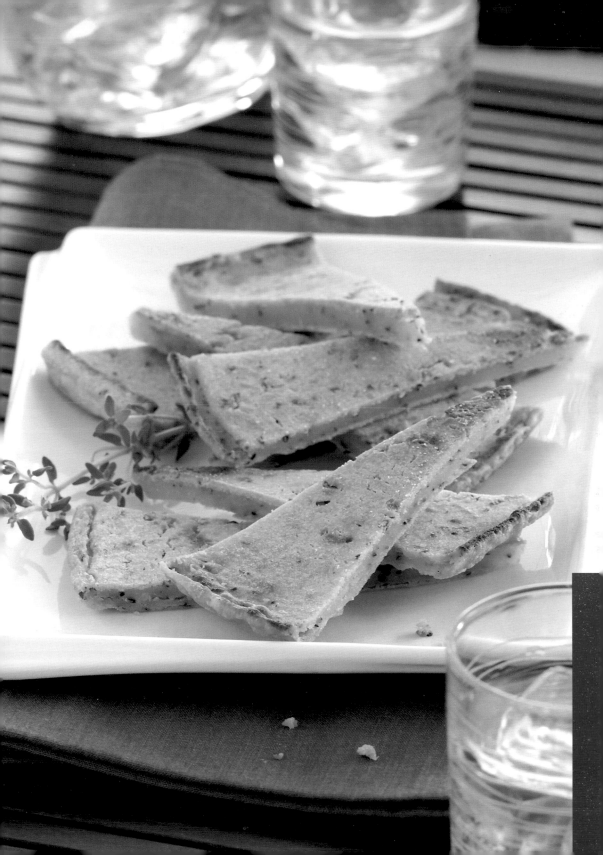

Kids' Pizzas

3 cups Gluten-Free Flour Blend for Breads (page 206)
2 packages (¼ ounce each) active dry yeast
2 teaspoons xanthan gum
1 teaspoon salt
1 cup warm water
¼ cup extra virgin olive oil
3 egg whites
1 tablespoon honey
1 teaspoon cider vinegar

Toppings
1 can (about 14 ounces) pizza sauce
Italian seasoning
1 package (about 3 ounces) sliced pepperoni
Shredded cheese (optional)

1. Preheat oven to 450°F. Line baking sheets or pizza pans with parchment paper.

2. Mix flour blend, yeast, xanthan gum and salt in large bowl. Whisk water, olive oil, egg whites, honey and vinegar in medium bowl. Beat wet ingredients into dry ingredients with electric mixer at low speed until combined. Add additional water by tablespoonfuls until batter is smooth and thick. Beat at medium-high speed 5 minutes, scraping bowl occasionally.

3. Transfer one sixth of dough to prepared pan. Spread dough into 5- or 6-inch circle using dampened fingers or back of oiled spoon, making crust thicker around edge to hold toppings. Repeat with remaining dough.

4. Bake 8 to 10 minutes or until crusts are lightly browned.* Top crusts with pizza sauce, Italian seasoning, pepperoni and cheese, if desired. Bake 2 to 5 minutes or until cheese melts. *Makes 6 (5- or 6-inch) pizzas*

To freeze pizza crusts for later use, allow them to cool, wrap well and store in the freezer for up to 3 months.

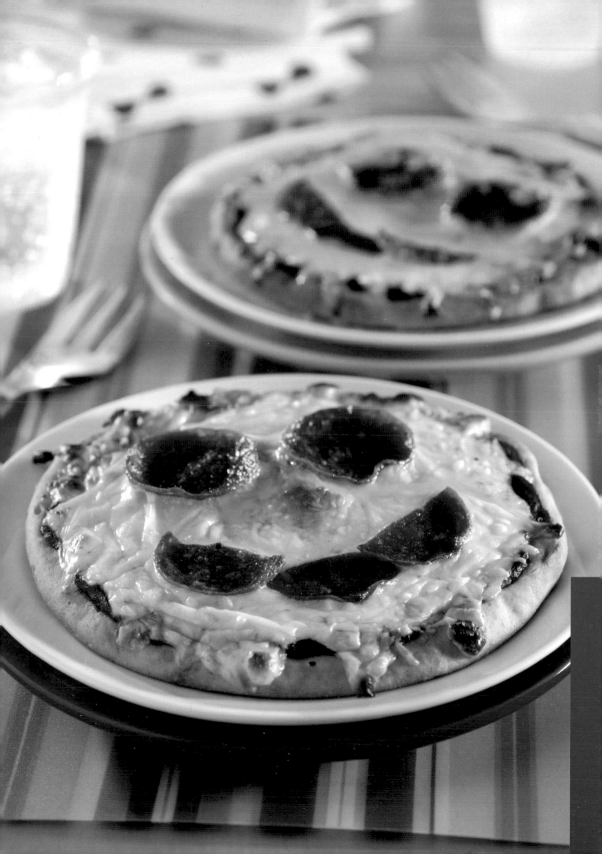

Olive & Herb Focaccia

3 cups Gluten-Free Flour Blend for Breads (page 206)
2 packages (¼ ounce each) active dry yeast
2 teaspoons xanthan gum
1 teaspoon salt
1 cup warm water
¼ cup extra virgin olive oil
3 egg whites
1 tablespoon honey
1 teaspoon cider vinegar

Toppings
1 cup chopped pitted kalamata olives
3 tablespoons chopped fresh rosemary leaves
2 tablespoons chopped fresh thyme
3 cloves garlic, minced
¼ cup extra virgin olive oil
Coarsely ground black pepper
¼ cup grated Romano cheese

1. Mix flour blend, yeast, xanthan gum and salt in large bowl. Whisk water, olive oil, egg whites, honey and vinegar in medium bowl. Beat wet ingredients into dry ingredients with electric mixer at low speed until combined. Add more water by tablespoonfuls, if needed, until batter is smooth, shiny and thick. Beat at medium-high speed 5 minutes, scraping bowl occasionally.

2. Preheat oven to 450°F. Line baking sheet with parchment paper or foil. Transfer half of dough to prepared baking sheet. Spread into 8-inch round about ½ inch thick using dampened hands. Repeat with remaining dough.

3. Let dough rest 20 minutes. Dimple top of dough with fingertips. Sprinkle with olives, rosemary, thyme and garlic. Drizzle with olive oil and sprinkle with pepper.

4. Bake about 15 minutes or until lightly browned. Sprinkle with cheese immediately. Cool on wire rack 2 or 3 minutes before slicing.

Makes 2 focaccia breads

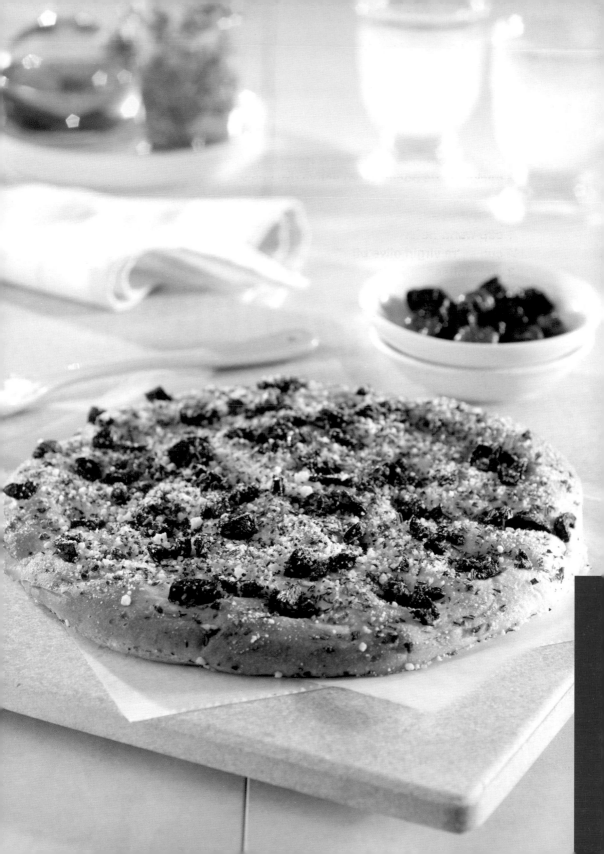

Gluten-Free Pizza

1¾ cups Gluten-Free Flour Blend for Breads (page 206)
1½ cups white rice flour, plus additional for work surface
  2 teaspoons sugar
  1 package (¼ ounce) active dry yeast
1½ teaspoons salt
1½ teaspoons Italian seasoning
  1 teaspoon baking powder
  ½ teaspoon xanthan gum
1¼ cups warm water (110°F)
  2 tablespoons olive oil
    Pizza sauce
    Toppings: fresh mozzarella cheese, sliced tomatoes, fresh basil, grated Parmesan cheese

1. Combine dry ingredients in large bowl. Add water in steady stream while beating with electric mixer at low speed until soft dough forms. Add olive oil; beat 2 minutes. Transfer to rice-floured surface and knead 2 minutes or until dough holds together in a smooth ball.

2. Place dough in oiled bowl; turn to coat. Cover; let rise in warm place 30 minutes. (Dough will increase in size but not double.)

3. Preheat oven to 400°F. Line pizza pan or baking sheet with foil. Punch down dough and transfer to center of prepared pan. Spread dough as thin as possible (about ⅛ inch thick) using dampened hands. Bake 5 to 7 minutes or until crust begins to color. (Crust may crack in spots.)

4. Spread pizza sauce over crust. Sprinkle with toppings. Bake 10 to 15 minutes or until cheese melts and pizza is cooked through.

Makes 4 to 6 servings

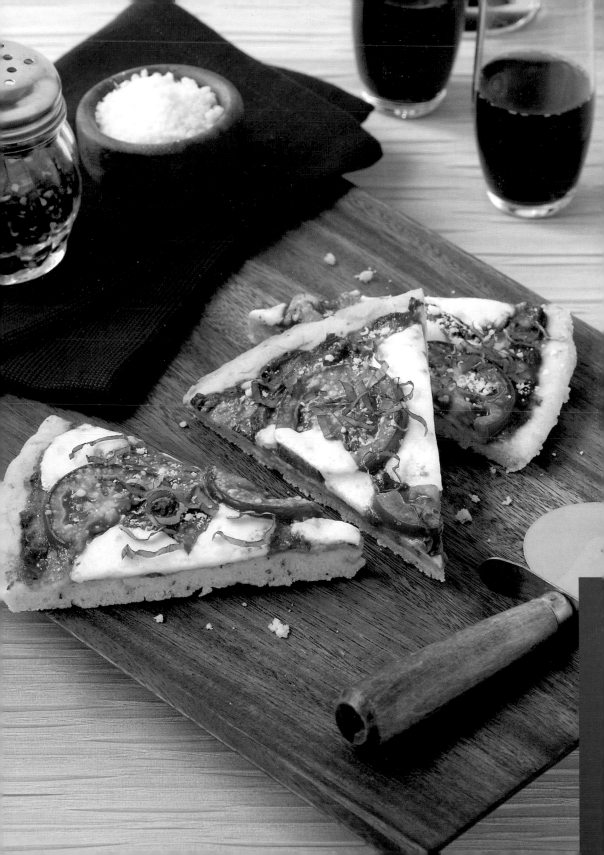

Slightly Sweet

Sweet Cherry Biscuits

   2 cups gluten-free biscuit baking mix
   ¼ cup sugar
   2 teaspoons baking powder
   ½ teaspoon salt
   ½ teaspoon crushed dried rosemary
   ½ cup (1 stick) unsalted butter, cut into small pieces
   ¾ cup milk
   ½ cup dried cherries, chopped

1. Preheat oven to 425°F. Combine baking mix, sugar, baking powder, salt and rosemary in large bowl. Cut in butter with pastry blender or two knives until mixture forms small crumbs. Stir in milk to form sticky batter. Stir in cherries.

2. Pat dough to 1-inch thickness on surface lightly dusted with baking mix. Cut out circles with 3-inch biscuit cutter. Place biscuits 1 inch apart on ungreased baking sheet. Bake about 15 minutes or until golden brown. Cool on wire rack 5 minutes before serving. *Makes about 10 biscuits*

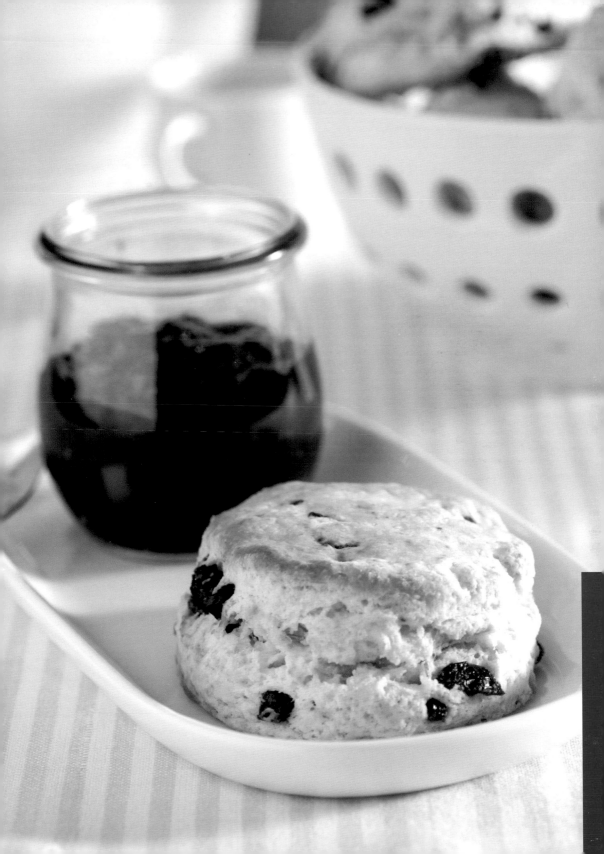

Lots o' Chocolate Bread

2 cups mini semisweet chocolate chips, divided

⅔ cup packed light brown sugar

½ cup (1 stick) butter

2 eggs

2½ cups Gluten-Free All-Purpose Flour Blend (page 206)*

1½ cups applesauce

1½ teaspoons vanilla

1½ teaspoons baking soda

1¼ teaspoons xanthan gum

1 teaspoon baking powder

½ teaspoon salt

1 tablespoon shortening (do not use butter, margarine, spread or oil)

Or use any all-purpose gluten-free flour blend that does not contain xanthan gum.

1. Preheat oven to 350°F. Grease 5 mini (5½×3-inch) loaf pans. Place 1 cup chocolate chips in small microwavable bowl. Microwave on HIGH 1 minute; stir. Microwave at 30-second intervals, stirring after each interval, until chocolate is melted.

2. Beat brown sugar and butter in large bowl with electric mixer at medium speed until creamy. Add melted chocolate and eggs; beat until well blended. Add flour blend, applesauce, vanilla, baking soda, xanthan gum, baking powder and salt; beat until well blended. Stir in ½ cup chocolate chips. Spoon batter evenly into prepared pans.

3. Bake 35 to 40 minutes or until centers crack and are dry to the touch. Cool in pans on wire racks 5 minutes. Remove from pans; cool completely.

4. Place remaining ½ cup chocolate chips and shortening in small microwavable bowl. Microwave on HIGH 1 minute; stir. Microwave at 30-second intervals, stirring after each interval, until chocolate is melted and mixture is smooth. Drizzle loaves with glaze; let stand until set.

Makes 5 mini loaves

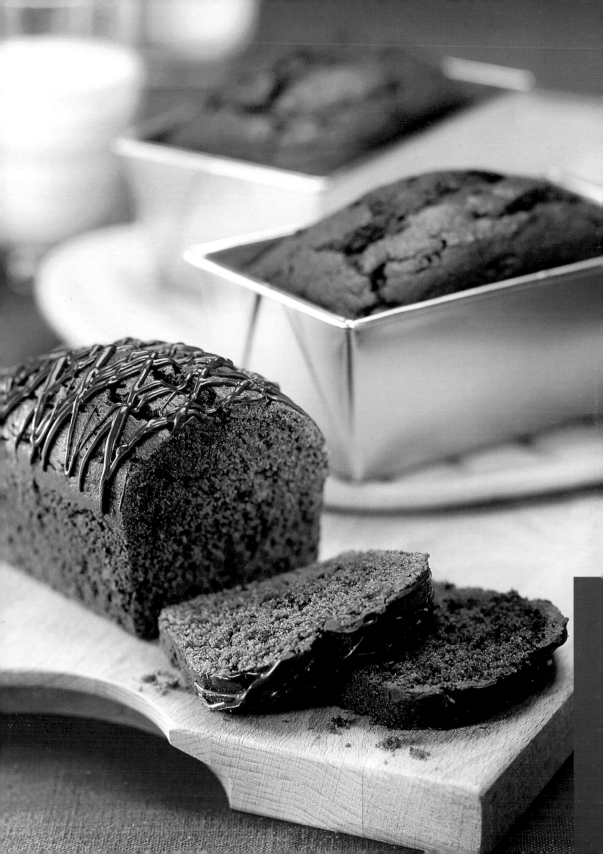

Orange-Lemon Citrus Bread

1¾ cups **Gluten-Free All-Purpose Flour Blend (page 206),* plus additional for pan**

¾ **cup sugar**

1 **tablespoon plus ½ teaspoon grated lemon peel, divided**

2 **teaspoons baking powder**

1 **teaspoon xanthan gum**

¼ **teaspoon salt**

1 **cup milk**

½ **cup vegetable oil**

1 **egg, beaten**

1 **teaspoon vanilla**

¼ **cup orange marmalade**

*Or use any all-purpose gluten-free flour blend that does not contain xanthan gum.

1. Preheat oven to 350°F. Grease and flour 9×5-inch loaf pan.

2. Whisk flour blend, sugar, 1 tablespoon lemon peel, baking powder, xanthan gum and salt in large bowl. Beat milk, oil, egg and vanilla in small bowl until well blended. Make well in flour mixture; pour in milk mixture and stir just until blended. (Batter will be thin.) Pour into prepared pan.

3. Bake 45 minutes or until toothpick inserted into center comes out clean. Cool in pan on wire rack 5 minutes.

4. Meanwhile, combine marmalade and remaining ½ teaspoon lemon peel in small microwavable bowl. Microwave on HIGH 15 seconds or until slightly melted. Remove bread from pan to wire rack; spread marmalade mixture evenly over top. Cool completely before serving.   *Makes 1 (9-inch) loaf*

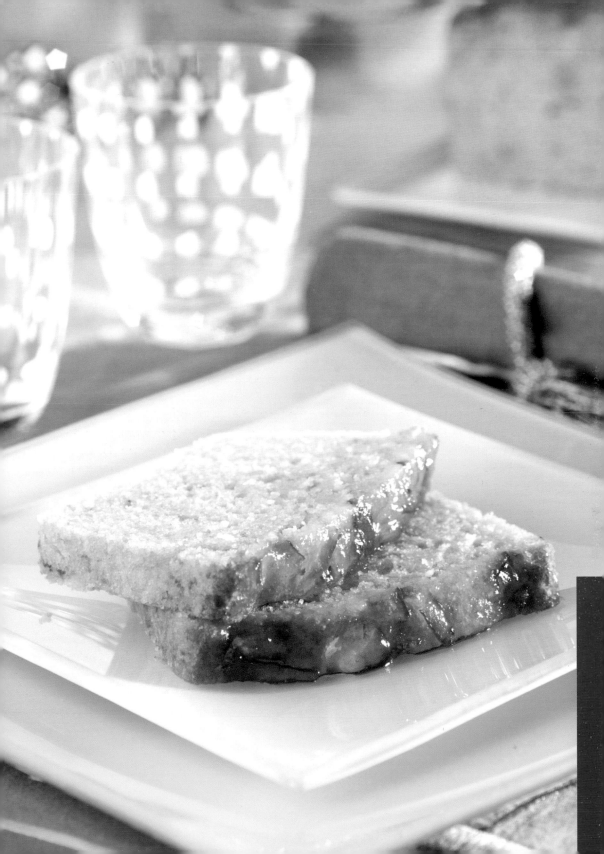

GF Graham Crackers

½ **cup sweet rice flour (mochiko), plus additional for work surface**
½ **cup sorghum flour**
½ **cup lightly packed brown sugar**
⅓ **cup tapioca flour**
½ **teaspoon baking soda**
½ **teaspoon salt**
¼ **cup (½ stick) dairy-free margarine**
2 **tablespoons plus 2 teaspoons soymilk or other milk**
2 **tablespoons honey**
1 **tablespoon vanilla**

1. Combine sweet rice flour, sorghum flour, brown sugar, tapioca flour, baking soda and salt in food processor. Pulse to combine, making sure brown sugar is free of lumps. Add margarine and pulse until coarse crumbs form.

2. Stir soymilk, honey and vanilla in measuring cup until honey dissolves. Pour into flour mixture and process until dough comes together. Dough will be very soft and sticky. Transfer dough to rice-floured surface; pat into rectangle. Wrap and refrigerate dough at least 4 hours or up to 2 days.

3. Preheat oven to 325°F. Cover work surface with parchment paper and generously flour parchment paper with rice flour.

4. Roll dough to ⅛-inch-thick rectangle on parchment using floured rolling pin. If dough becomes too sticky, return to refrigerator or freezer for several minutes. Transfer dough on parchment to baking sheet. Score dough into cracker shapes (do not cut all the way through). Prick dough in rows with tines of fork. Place baking sheet in freezer for 5 to 10 minutes or in refrigerator for 15 to 20 minutes.

5. Transfer cold crackers directly to oven; bake 25 minutes or until firm and a shade darker. Transfer parchment to wire rack to cool. Cut crackers apart when cooled slightly.   *Makes about 1 dozen crackers*

S'mores: Place chocolate squares on GF Graham Crackers. Top with toasted marshmallows and additional GF Graham Crackers.

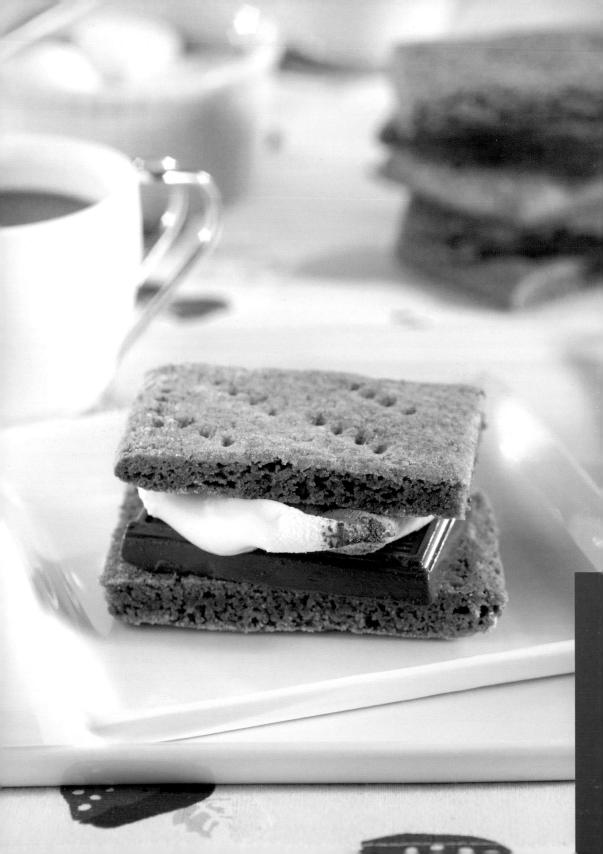

Zucchini Bread

2½ **cups Gluten-Free All-Purpose Flour Blend (page 206)***

⅔ **cup packed brown sugar**

½ **cup teff flour**

⅓ **cup granulated sugar**

1 **tablespoon baking powder**

2 **teaspoons ground cinnamon**

1 **teaspoon baking soda**

1 **teaspoon salt**

¾ **teaspoon xanthan gum**

¼ **teaspoon ground allspice**

¼ **teaspoon ground nutmeg**

¼ **teaspoon ground cardamom**

1¼ **cups milk**

2 **eggs**

¼ **cup canola oil**

1 **teaspoon vanilla**

1½ **cups grated zucchini, squeezed dry**

*Or use any all-purpose gluten-free flour blend that does not contain xanthan gum.

1. Preheat oven to 350°F. Grease 9×5-inch loaf pan.

2. Combine flour blend, brown sugar, teff flour, granulated sugar, baking powder, cinnamon, baking soda, salt, xanthan gum, allspice, nutmeg and cardamom in large bowl.

3. Whisk milk, eggs, oil and vanilla in medium bowl.

4. Make well in center of dry ingredients; stir in milk mixture. Stir in zucchini. Pour into prepared pan. Bake 1 hour or until toothpick inserted into center comes out almost clean. Cool in pan on wire rack 5 minutes. Remove from pan; cool completely.   *Makes 1 (9-inch) loaf*

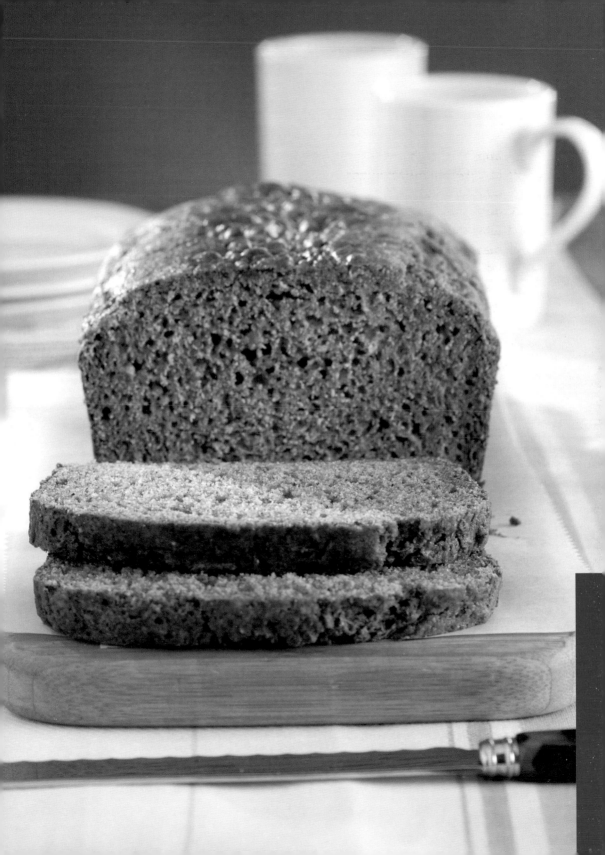

Chocolate Chip Scones

2 cups Gluten-Free All-Purpose Flour Blend (page 206),* plus additional for work surface

¼ cup sugar

2½ teaspoons baking powder

¾ teaspoon salt

¾ teaspoon xanthan gum

½ teaspoon baking soda

1 cup semisweet chocolate chips, divided

½ cup (1 stick) cold butter, cut into small pieces

½ cup plain yogurt

¾ cup milk

*Or use any all-purpose gluten-free flour blend that does not contain xanthan gum.

1. Preheat oven to 425°F.

2. Combine flour blend, sugar, baking powder, salt, xanthan gum and baking soda in large bowl. Add ½ cup chocolate chips and toss to combine.

3. Cut butter into flour mixture with pastry blender or two knives until coarse crumbs form. Stir yogurt into milk in small bowl.

4. Gradually add yogurt mixture to flour mixture, stirring just until dough begins to form. (You may not need all of yogurt mixture.) Transfer to surface sprinkled with flour blend. Knead 5 or 6 times until dough holds together. Divide into 3 pieces.

5. Pat each dough piece into circle about ½ inch thick. Cut each circle into 6 wedges with floured knife. Transfer scones to baking sheet, spacing 2 inches apart.

6. Bake 10 to 14 minutes or until lightly browned. Cool on wire rack. Meanwhile, place remaining ½ cup chocolate chips in microwavable bowl. Microwave on HIGH 1 minute or until melted. Drizzle over scones.

Makes 18 scones

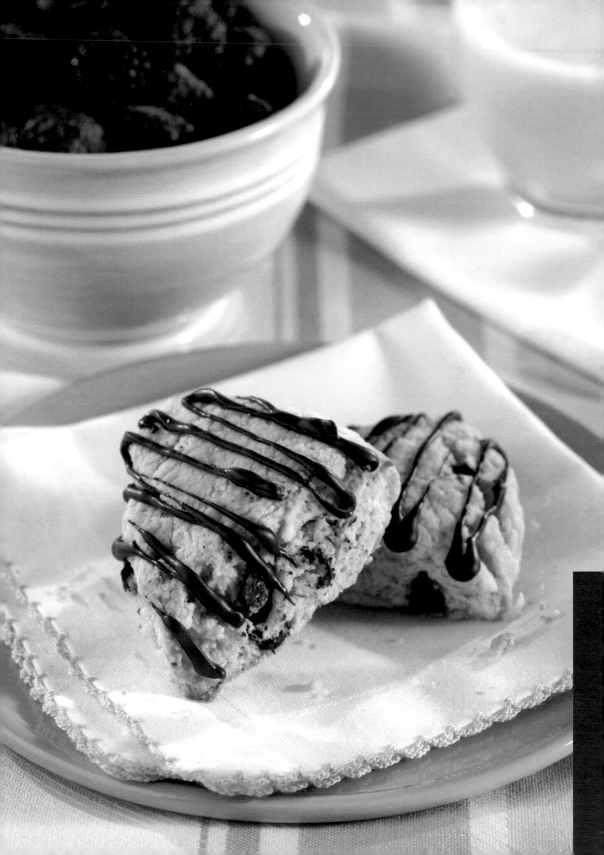

Date & Walnut Bread

- **1 cup boiling water**
- **¾ cup chopped pitted dates (8 to 10 Medjool dates)**
- **½ cup brown rice flour**
- **½ cup almond flour**
- **½ cup cornstarch**
- **¼ cup tapioca flour**
- **¼ cup gluten-free oat flour**
- **1 tablespoon baking powder**
- **1 teaspoon xanthan gum**
- **1 teaspoon baking soda**
- **½ teaspoon salt**
- **½ teaspoon ground cardamom**
- **1 cup packed brown sugar**
- **¼ cup canola oil**
- **2 eggs**
- **1 teaspoon vanilla**
- **1 cup walnuts, coarsely chopped**

1. Preheat oven to 350°F. Grease 9×5-inch loaf pan. Pour boiling water over dates in small bowl; set aside until softened and cooled.

2. Whisk brown rice flour, almond flour, cornstarch, tapioca flour, oat flour, baking powder, xanthan gum, baking soda, salt and cardamom in medium bowl.

3. Stir brown sugar and oil in large bowl. Add eggs, one at a time, beating well after each addition. Stir in vanilla and dates with soaking water. Add flour mixture; stir until combined. Stir in walnuts.

4. Spoon into prepared pan. Bake 50 to 55 minutes or until toothpick inserted into center comes out clean. (Check after 35 minutes and cover with foil to prevent overbrowning if necessary.) Cool in pan on wire rack 5 minutes. Remove from pan; cool completely. *Makes 1 (9-inch) loaf*

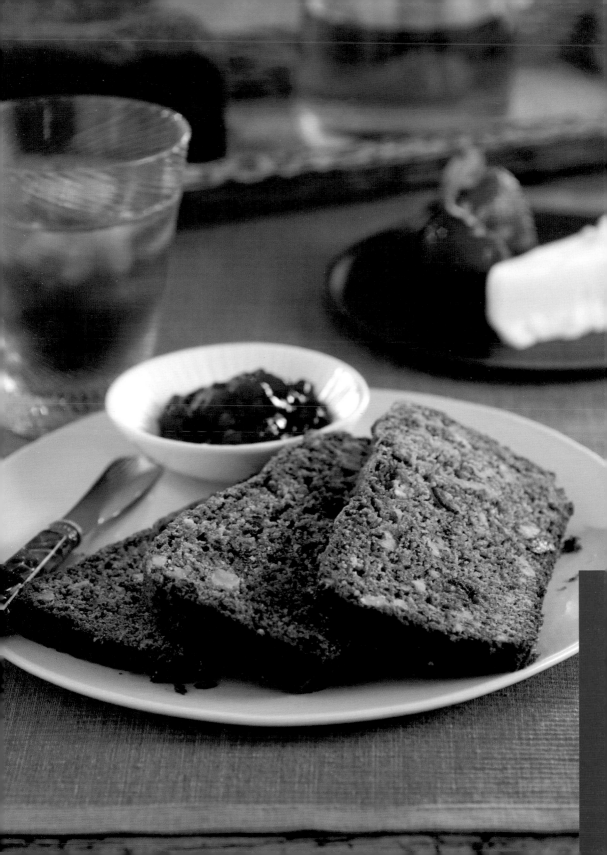

Chocolate Chip Elvis Bread

2½ cups Gluten-Free All-Purpose Flour Blend (page 206)*

½ cup granulated sugar

½ cup packed brown sugar

1 tablespoon baking powder

1 teaspoon xanthan gum

¾ teaspoon salt

1 cup mashed ripe bananas (about 2 large)

1 cup milk

¾ cup peanut butter

¼ cup vegetable oil

1 egg

1 teaspoon vanilla

1 cup semisweet chocolate chips

Or use any all-purpose gluten-free flour blend that does not contain xanthan gum.

1. Preheat oven to 350°F. Spray 4 mini (5½×3-inch) loaf pans with nonstick cooking spray.

2. Combine flour blend, granulated sugar, brown sugar, baking powder, xanthan gum and salt in large bowl; mix well. Beat bananas, milk, peanut butter, oil, egg and vanilla in medium bowl until well blended. Add banana mixture and chocolate chips to flour mixture; stir just until moistened. Pour into prepared pans.

3. Bake 40 minutes or until toothpick inserted into centers comes out clean. Cool in pans on wire racks 5 minutes. Remove from pans; cool completely.

Makes 4 mini loaves

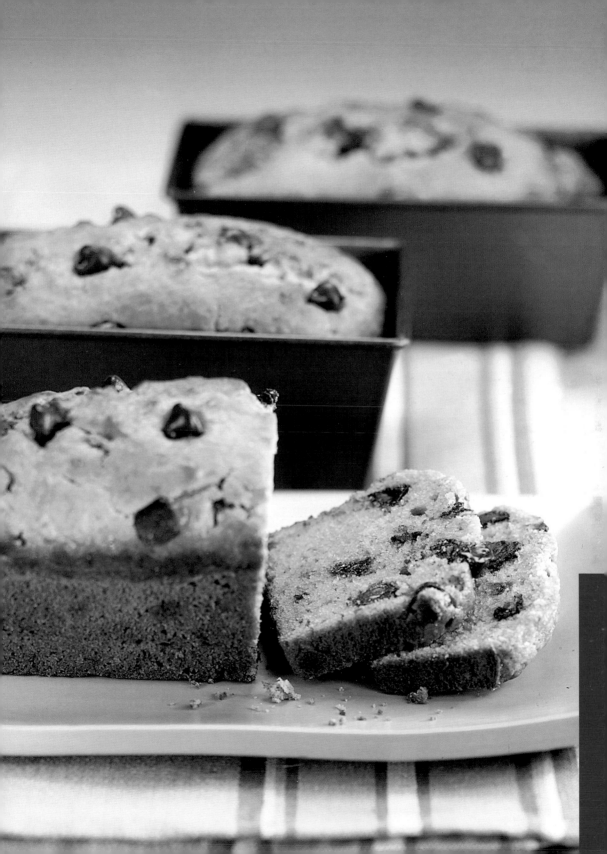

Apricot Cranberry Scones

2 cups **Gluten-Free All-Purpose Flour Blend (page 206),* plus additional for work surface**

¼ **cup sugar**

2½ **teaspoons baking powder**

¾ **teaspoon salt**

¾ **teaspoon xanthan gum**

½ **teaspoon baking soda**

¼ **cup chopped dried apricots**

¼ **cup dried cranberries**

½ **cup (1 stick) cold butter, cut into small pieces**

½ **cup plain yogurt**

¾ **cup milk**

*Or use any all-purpose gluten-free flour blend that does not contain xanthan gum.

1. Preheat oven to 425°F.

2. Combine flour blend, sugar, baking powder, salt, xanthan gum and baking soda in large bowl. Add apricots and cranberries; toss to combine.

3. Cut butter into flour mixture with pastry blender or two knives until coarse crumbs form. Stir yogurt into milk in small bowl or large measuring cup until combined.

4. Gradually add wet ingredients to dry ingredients, stirring just until dough begins to form. (You may not need all of yogurt mixture.) Transfer to surface sprinkled with flour blend. Knead 5 or 6 times until dough holds together.

5. Pat dough into circle about ½ inch thick. Cut into 2-inch circles with floured biscuit cutter. Transfer scones to baking sheet, spacing 2 inches apart. Press together remaining dough and cut additional scones.

6. Bake 10 to 14 minutes or until lightly browned. Cool on wire rack.

Makes about 15 scones

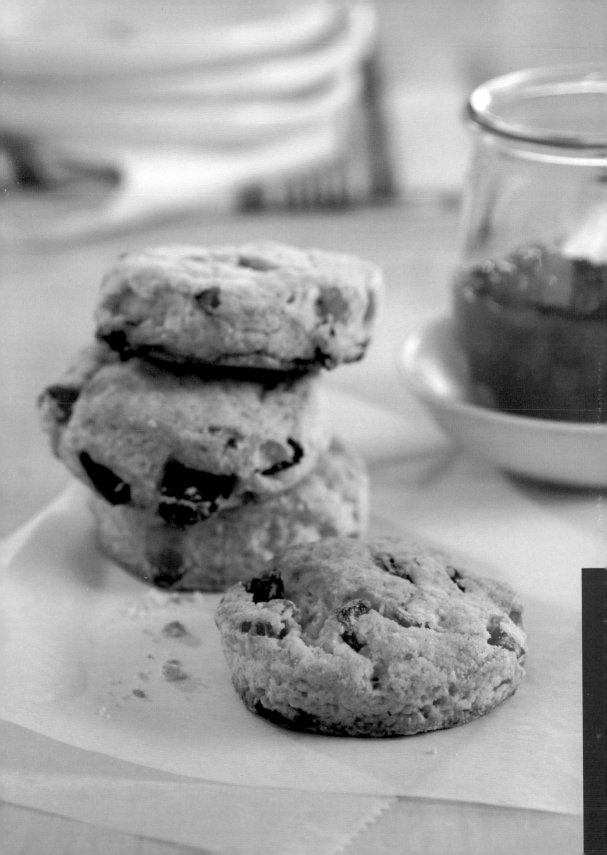

Applesauce-Spice Bread

1½ cups Gluten-Free All-Purpose Flour Blend (page 206)*
1½ cups unsweetened applesauce
¾ cup packed light brown sugar
½ cup shortening
1 teaspoon vanilla
1 teaspoon baking soda
1 teaspoon ground cinnamon
¾ teaspoon xanthan gum
½ teaspoon baking powder
¼ teaspoon salt
¼ teaspoon ground nutmeg
½ cup toasted chopped walnuts
½ cup raisins
Powdered sugar

*Or use any all-purpose gluten-free flour blend that does not contain xanthan gum.

1. Preheat oven to 350°F. Spray 9-inch square baking pan with nonstick cooking spray.

2. Beat flour blend, applesauce, brown sugar, shortening, vanilla, baking soda, cinnamon, xanthan gum, baking powder, salt and nutmeg in large bowl with electric mixer at low speed 30 seconds. Beat at high speed 3 minutes. Stir in walnuts and raisins. Pour into prepared pan.

3. Bake 30 minutes or until toothpick inserted into center comes out clean. Cool in pan on wire rack. Sprinkle with powdered sugar before serving.

Makes 9 servings

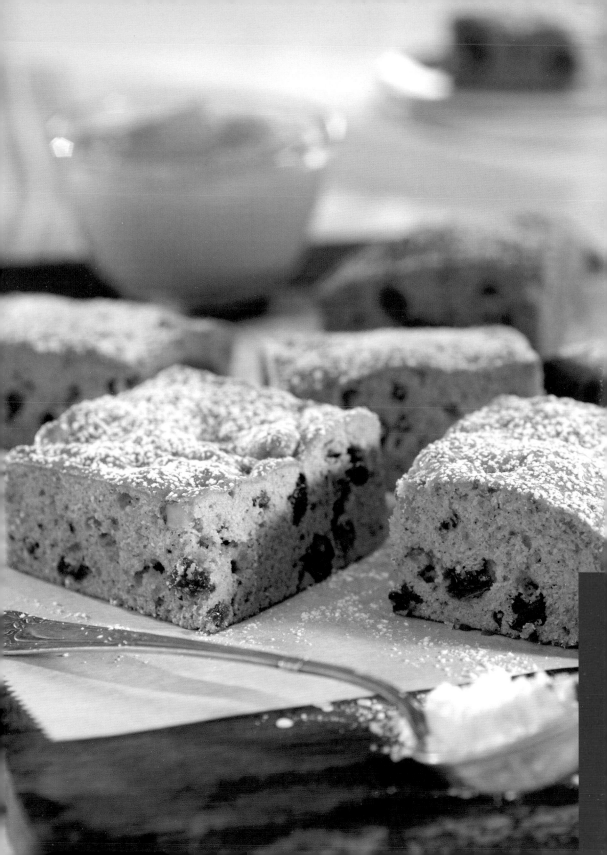

METRIC CONVERSION CHART

VOLUME MEASUREMENTS (dry)

1/8 teaspoon = 0.5 mL
1/4 teaspoon = 1 mL
1/2 teaspoon = 2 mL
3/4 teaspoon = 4 mL
1 teaspoon = 5 mL
1 tablespoon = 15 mL
2 tablespoons = 30 mL
1/4 cup = 60 mL
1/3 cup = 75 mL
1/2 cup = 125 mL
2/3 cup = 150 mL
3/4 cup = 175 mL
1 cup = 250 mL
2 cups = 1 pint = 500 mL
3 cups = 750 mL
4 cups = 1 quart = 1 L

VOLUME MEASUREMENTS (fluid)

1 fluid ounce (2 tablespoons) = 30 mL
4 fluid ounces (1/2 cup) = 125 mL
8 fluid ounces (1 cup) = 250 mL
12 fluid ounces (1 1/2 cups) = 375 mL
16 fluid ounces (2 cups) = 500 mL

WEIGHTS (mass)

1/2 ounce = 15 g
1 ounce = 30 g
3 ounces = 90 g
4 ounces = 120 g
8 ounces = 225 g
10 ounces = 285 g
12 ounces = 360 g
16 ounces = 1 pound = 450 g

DIMENSIONS

1/16 inch = 2 mm
1/8 inch = 3 mm
1/4 inch = 6 mm
1/2 inch = 1.5 cm
3/4 inch = 2 cm
1 inch = 2.5 cm

OVEN TEMPERATURES

250°F = 120°C
275°F = 140°C
300°F = 150°C
325°F = 160°C
350°F = 180°C
375°F = 190°C
400°F = 200°C
425°F = 220°C
450°F = 230°C

BAKING PAN SIZES

Utensil	Size in Inches/Quarts	Metric Volume	Size in Centimeters
Baking or	8×8×2	2 L	20×20×5
Cake Pan	9×9×2	2.5 L	23×23×5
(square or	12×8×2	3 L	30×20×5
rectangular)	13×9×2	3.5 L	33×23×5
Loaf Pan	8×4×3	1.5 L	20×10×7
	9×5×3	2 L	23×13×7
Round Layer	8×1½	1.2 L	20×4
Cake Pan	9×1½	1.5 L	23×4
Pie Plate	8×1¼	750 mL	20×3
	9×1¼	1 L	23×3
Baking Dish	1 quart	1 L	—
or Casserole	1½ quart	1.5 L	—
	2 quart	2 L	—